The 60-Second EMT
RAPID BLS/ALS ASSESSMENT, DIAGNOSIS & TRIAGE

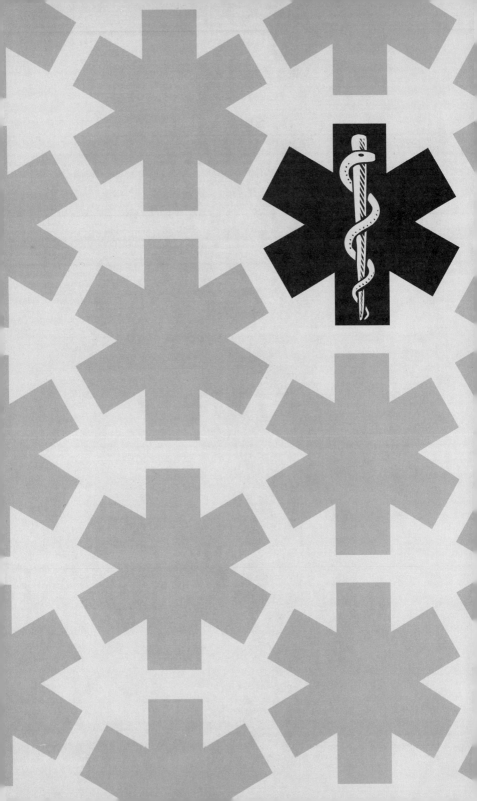

The 60-Second EMT

Rapid BLS/ALS Assessment, Diagnosis & Triage

SECOND EDITION

Gideon Bosker, MD, FACEP
Donald Weins, MD, FACEP
Michael Sequeira, MD, FACEP

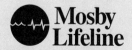

St. Louis Baltimore Boston Carlsbad Chicago Naples New York Philadelphia Portland
London Madrid Mexico City Singapore Sydney Tokyo Toronto Wiesbaden

Publisher: David Dusthimer
Executive Editor: Claire Merrick
Editor: Rina Steinhauer
Developmental Editor: Harold Cohen
Assistant Editor: Melissa Blair
Project Manager: Chris Baumle
Production Editor: David Orzechowski
Designer Manager: Nancy McDonald
Cover Illustrator: Chris Gall

Second Edition

Copyright © 1996 by Mosby—Year Book, Inc.

Printed in the United States of America
Composition by University Graphics, Inc.
Printing/Binding by R.R. Donnelley & Sons Company

Mosby—Year Book, Inc.
11830 Westline Industrial Drive
St. Louis, Missouri 63146

Library of Congress Cataloging-in-Publication Data

Bosker, Gideon.
    The 60-second EMT: rapid BLS/ALS assessment, diagnosis & triage/
Gideon Bosker, Donald Weins, Michael Sequeira.--2nd ed.
        p.   cm.
    Includes index.
    ISBN 0-8016-7812-9 (alk. paper)
    1. Emergency medicine. 2. Emergency medical technicians.
I. Weins, Donald.   II. Sequeira, Michael.   III. Title.
    [DNLM: 1. Emergency Medical Services. 2. Emergencies.
3. Emergency Medical Technicians. WX 215 B743z 1995]
RC86.7.B675 1996
616.02'5--dc20
DNLM/DLC
for Library of Congress   95-30731
                                                            CIP

98 99 00 01 / 9 8 7 6 5 4 3

Publisher Acknowledgements

The editors wish to acknowledge and thank the following reviewers. Their comments were enlightening and invaluable in helping develop the expanded second edition of this book.

Jerry Bardwell, NREMT-P
Claremont, New Hampshire

Ann Bellows, RN, REMT-P
Las Cruces, New Mexico

Jo Ann Cobble, NREMT-P
Jacksonville, Arkansas

William Raynovich, NREMT-P
Kenhorst, Pennsylvania

Tom Vines, EMT-D
Red Lodge, Montana

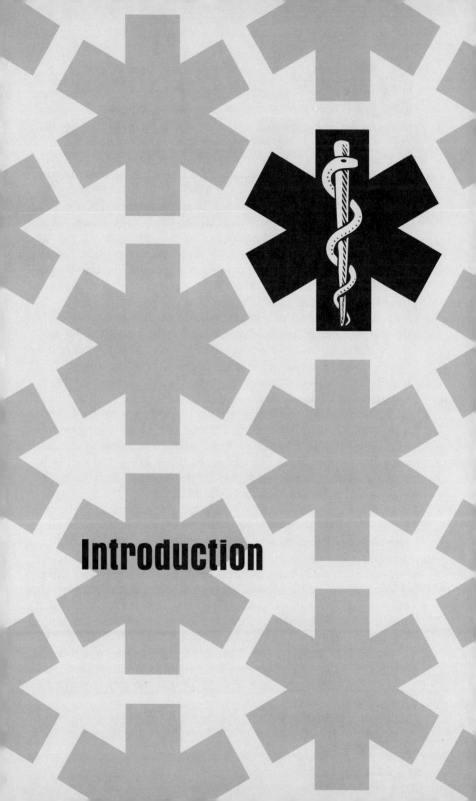

Introduction

he *60-Second EMT: Rapid BSL/ALS Assessment, Diagnosis & Triage* provides a thoughtful, critical, decision-making approach to the practice of prehospital medical care. Presenting a number of common emergency situations—from syncope, chest pain, and coma to multiple trauma, toxicologic emergencies, and respiratory failure—this book intertwines the narrative intrigue of a lively quest story (the search for the "60-Second" EMT) with the author's hard-won clinical knowledge gleaned from years of prehospital experience. Because rapid, accurate assessment is the key to the best prehospital management, special attention is given to the development of a systematic approach to prehospital evaluation based on the clinical history, the primary and secondary survey, the mechanism of injury, and the acuteness of the patient's condition.

Since publication of the first edition of *The 60-Second EMT*, the requirements for assessment and intervention skills have evolved dramatically. Over the past few years, trauma center designations and increasing hospital specialization according to clinical service have necessitated improved assessment skills for Emergency Medical Technicians (EMTs). EMTs must direct patients to institutions best equipped to meet their needs. In addition, because of an irreversible demographic shift, today's prehospital care providers transport more geriatric patients. Prehospital care demands increased expertise in recognizing and caring for patients with diseases common to the elderly such as stroke, myocardial infarction, and fall-related trauma.

Perhaps most important, prehospital care providers are becoming an integral therapeutic arm of the entire Emergency Medical Services (EMS) system. Many communities have integrated immediate care by EMTs into thrombolytic treatment protocols for patients with acute myocardial infarction. To address this expansion of EMT care for coronary artery disease, this edition of *The 60-Second EMT* includes state-of-the-art protocols for assessment, stabilization, thrombolytic therapy, and other lifesaving measures for acute myocardial infarction. New treatment options have emerged also for acute cerebrovascular disorders. Accordingly, this edition includes several new algorithms for stroke and coma assessment that have been issued by the Neurological Stroke Association.

Finally, as in any profession, the world of prehospital care is constantly evolving under the influence of new therapies. EMT practitioners, as they gain experience, find themselves challenged with greater assessment and care responsibilities. This edition contains more than 50 new tables, side bars, and boxed material to help refine, upgrade, and expand assessment and care capabilities of EMTs.

This new edition of *The 60-Second EMT* is written to provide an educational and entertaining, yet rigorous and comprehensive approach for EMTs at all levels—from EMT-B to EMT-P—who wish to practice effective prehospital care. Vignettes with dialogue between the narrator and EMTs encountered in the quest to find the "60-Second" EMT are intended to simulate the kinds of questions and concerns that EMTs and paramedics have consistently raised. In addition, we have developed each module using history-taking issues, diagnostic concepts, and therapeutic skills that will stimulate EMTs and paramedics to develop a "special instinct" for prehospital assessment and triage. The goal of this book is to inform prehospital care providers and guide them on the road to becoming "60-second" EMTs.

The prehospital encounters in *The 60-Second EMT* will be of interest to every EMT who intends to improve his or her skills, knowledge, and professional expertise. In this vein, we present systematic assessment methods, data gathering techniques, and diagnostic approaches that address critical prehospital concerns of EMTs and paramedics. The basic life support (BLS) portions of the clinical encounters have been constructed so that the assessment skills are advanced enough to stimulate EMTs, yet the advanced life support (ALS) skills and assessment techniques present enough depth and detail to interest and educate paramedics.

Although the therapeutic interventions sometimes fall within the scope of paramedic/ALS practice, we believe that it is important for EMTs at all levels to follow a course of action from beginning to end—from assessment to treatment—even if some of the therapeutic approaches fall outside the scope of their practice. As always, there is no better way to learn than to be exposed to a patient's entire prehospital course.

The book is organized in the form of a quest story. It can be read at one sitting or in several sessions. The first chapter introduces the reader to Jerry Donnelly, a (fictional) highly respected EMT who has created, developed, and mastered the skills and assessment techniques of the "60-second" program. In the second chapter, the reader will become familiar with the concept of the *Golden*

Minute, the crucial unit of time in which EMTs interview, assess, and determine a productive course of action in a prehospital setting.

After the first two, the book's chapters are organized around a specific clinical module: chest pain, trauma, respiratory distress, etc. They are divided into complementary parts: the first section is written in the format of a dialogue encounter with an EMT co-worker of Donnelly's, who offers his or her view of some specific aspect of Donnelly's 60-second approach to prehospital care. The second section distills the information gleaned from this conversation into an easy-to-use guide called the "60-Second Capsule."

Using a creative and innovative approach, *The 60-Second EMT* focuses on state-of-the-art prehospital clinical skills, assessment strategies, and treatment protocols and the challenge these create. Our hope is that after reading this book, EMTs who wish to maintain the highest standards of care will gain a new appreciation for assessment and triage skills. The book is intended to teach EMTs to (1) detect at once diagnostic clues that usually take much longer to recognize; (2) select and institute appropriate, oftentimes life saving, therapies within moments; (3) proceed quickly through established EMT algorithms and treatment protocols; (4) take capsule histories that provide active approaches to prehospital care; (5) learn when to use the "Contemplative History-Oriented Response" (CHOR) and when to use the "Fast Action Saves Time" (FAST) track in prehospital evaluation; and, finally, (6) decrease reaction time, that is, reduce the critical period between assessment and intervention. These skills are the vital signs of outstanding prehospital care. Now, sit back and enjoy the story . . . .

Gideon Bosker, M.D., F.A.C.E.P.
Portland, Oregon 1995

Contents

1

The Search for the 60-Second EMT

Two years before my meeting with Jerry Donnelly, I learned through the Emergency Medical Services (EMS) grapevine that Jerry was something of a celebrity in the Emergency Medical Technician (EMT) world. His expertise in rapidly assessing patients had earned him a reputation as the "60-Second" EMT. That was enough to pique my interest and start me on my quest. But I became even more excited when I learned from a number of EMTs whom I respected that Donnelly was not only "quick on his feet," but also had a reputation for being very accurate and precise in his prehospital evaluations. We all know that combining speed and accuracy in assessment is the key to successful stabilization, management, and triage of patients in the field.

> Combining speed and accuracy in assessment is the key to successful stabilization, management, and triage of patients in the field.

In fact, Donnelly was so good at what he did that over the past 10 years, he had risen to almost guru-like status within his EMS community. He was a hospital-based EMT in a large metropolitan area. His duties as a practicing EMT, instructor, and administrator had brought him into contact with physicians, nurses, first-responders and others from all components of the EMS system. Praise for Donnelly was never in short supply. Everyone said that he was one of the nicest people you would ever meet . . . and modest, too. Apparently, there were good reasons for his attaining such an amazing reputation.

Donnelly's 60-Second EMT program had been praised by a number of instructors as a new and creative approach to prehospital assessment. From what I had heard, Donnelly had developed this field assessment program over a number of years with the help of several other EMTs in the community. Most of his collaborators were considered the shining stars in the community's EMS system.

Those EMTs and paramedics who have used the 60-second approach—and most who know about it do use it—give the method high marks for teaching prehospital providers at all levels a systematic approach to diagnosing and triaging life-threatening emergencies during the first minute of a patient encounter. These EMTs claim that the 60-second program has helped them develop a "sixth sense" for assessing and managing prehospital emergencies. On the basis of my own experiences in the field, I know that a special "touch" for diagnosing patients does not come easily. After years of professional practice, even the best EMTs find that they are still learning clinical skills the hard way—out in the field, by trial and error.

At its beginning, one of the main purposes of the 60-Second EMT Program was to teach these hard-won "pearls," learned from years of experience and research, in a systematic way, so that EMTs would have a heightened awareness for unusual ways in which life-threatening illnesses and traumatic emergencies appear. Also, they would know how to piece together relevant historical information and clinical findings. "When it comes to assessment skills, we're starting more and more to feel like we have to be able to diagnose like doctors," is the way one experienced EMT put it. "There is no question that the 60-Second EMT Program has been instrumental in giving us the tools to improve ourselves and move in that direction."

That was the kind of confidence Donnelly's approach offered. "I can focus on the patient's most likely diagnosis earlier in my primary survey and implement my treatment protocols faster than I've ever been able to," one EMT confided. Others mentioned that their ability to communicate case histories and make oral presentations had been upgraded significantly by the 60-Second EMT Program.

In short, I heard nothing but glowing reports. Yet the more I heard people rave about the 60-Second EMT, the more I began to wonder: Can EMTs and paramedics really obtain all of the information they need to know about a patient within the first minute of their encounter? It just does not seem possible.

In fact, it was not. And Jerry Donnelly was the first person to tell me so when we finally met.

"The 60-Second EMT *can't* complete all the assessment and management interventions required of each prehospital encounter in the first minute," he explained. "That's simply not possible."

"Then what can he or she do? And what's special about your approach?" I asked.

"I'm glad you asked me to clarify this point," Jerry said amicably. "What the 60-Second EMT *can* do is diagnose rapidly and therefore make appropriate interventions when they are likely to do the most good. The 60-Second EMT pursues a productive line of questioning very early in the patient encounter. He or she can take a quick look at the scene, interview the patient, and know exactly where to start on treatment protocols. My skilled students can accomplish this within the critical Golden Minute.''

''That's impressive.'' I said.

''You see, it is within the first 60 seconds that initial impressions are so often made,'' continued Donnelly, ''and the purpose of the 60-second program is to steer the EMT toward the correct diagnosis as soon as possible. You have to be able to make the correct assessment before beginning treatment.''

> It is within the first 60 seconds that initial impressions are so often made.

''How are those initial impressions formed, and how do you sift out diagnostic clues that shed light on a case?'' I asked.

''They're formed on the basis of many different bits of information,'' Donnelly answered. ''It begins with the dispatcher's call, which can give the EMT a very rough sketch of what kind of problem the patient is having. This period of time is crucial because the 60-second clock hasn't started to tick. I encourage 60-Second EMTs to consider diagnostic possibilities and interventions en route *to the patient*. This is 'free clinical time' that allows you to tune into the general problem and prepare for intervention.''

Donnelly's point was well taken. He seemed to be saying that the 60-second approach heightened the EMT's awareness even before he arrived at the scene. But I still wanted to know what the 60-Second EMT program could offer someone like me—an EMT with a passion for excellence and a constant search for ways to refine my knowledge and skills.

Jerry continued. ''You see, the 60-second approach is designed to improve history-taking techniques and shorten the amount of time between the moment the EMT encounters the patient and the moment he or she makes his or her first therapeutic intervention. My experience is that this period can be a minute or less.''

> 60-Second EMTs should consider diagnostic possibilities and interventions en route to the patient.

''So you're saying the 60-Second EMT program is something like a catalyst? That it speeds up the reaction time?''

''Exactly,'' Donnelly said. ''Using improved assessment techniques during the first minute of patient encounter, the EMT can ''speedskate'' through established treatment protocols and algorithms. Prehospital care providers have to assess and diagnose before they treat. That's where the 60-Second EMT comes in.''

I settled in for a long afternoon of questions and answers. I thought it would be just a matter of letting Donnelly tell his story.

"So tell me, Jerry, why do they call you the '60-Second EMT'?" I asked.

Jerry, with the mystical look in his eyes that so many people had told me about, said shyly, "Because it's a system based on speed; the best way to understand it is to go and find out for yourself."

Using improved assessment techniques during the first minute of patient encounter, the EMT can "speedskate" through established treatment protocols and algorithms.

He reached into a drawer and pulled out a stapled lecture entitled *The Golden Minute*.

"Here you go," he said, handing me a copy. "This is as good a place as any to start your research."

"Great," I said. "I'll take this home and read it tonight. Tell you what, I'll come back tomorrow and then you can tell me *why* they call you the '60-Second EMT.' "

"I wish I could help you there, but I just can't," he explained. What I suggest is that you go and talk with my co-workers. Talk with the EMTs and paramedics I've worked with and let them tell you about the cases we've handled together. They'll tell you the way I approach and think about cases. I think that's where you'll get your answer."

It was obvious that Jerry was not going to budge. Quickly leafing through *The Golden Minute*, I realized that I had some homework to do before I began my quest to understand the 60-Second EMT.

"Thanks for everything, Jerry," I said as I made for the door. "Maybe I'll come back someday after I get my questions answered."

"You do that," he said with a big grin as he opened the door. "Good luck."

I brought *The Golden Minute* back to my sleeping quarters and started reading. It intrigued me from the outset. I could see that Donnelly had not just developed the laundry list of problems and solutions that you see in so many textbooks; he had developed a *system*. A strategy. That was the beauty of it. I was so excited that I woke up Forrest Mather, my partner, who was asleep in the top bunk.

"Get up, Forrest! You've got to read this Golden Minute lecture. It's written by Jerry Donnelly, the 60-Second EMT."

Still fuzzy with sleep, Forrest said, "Golden minute . . . you've got it right. That's exactly the amount of sleep I've had all night! Now, get off my back would you?"

"No, just listen to me; you've got to read this."

With the help of an ice bag and a crutch, I managed to pry the reluctant Forrest out of bed. We studied *The Golden Minute* together late into the night. This is what we found. . . .

2

The Golden Minute

Rapid Diagnosis and Assessment Skills for the 60-Second EMT
by Jerry Donnelly, EMT

I. The Golden Minute

A. What is the "Golden Minute"?
1. The "Golden Minute" is to the 60-Second EMT what the "Golden Hour" is to the emergency department physician: **The crucial unit of time in which to interview, assess, inspect, and determine a likely course of action in the prehospital setting.**

B. The Five Golden Rules
1. Stay calm.
2. Use a systematic approach to interview and assess the patient.
3. Assume the worst.
4. Look and inquire beyond the obvious.
5. Use protocols when warranted and be aggressive with stabilization.

C. The Golden Minute Objectives
1. Detect diagnostic clues early in the prehospital encounter.
2. Elicit capsule histories that yield action-oriented approaches to prehospital care.
3. Move rapidly down established EMT algorithms and standardized treatment protocols.
4. Select and institute appropriate, oftentimes life saving, therapy within moments.

D. Golden Minute Pathways
One of the following pathways usually will be more appropriate than the other. Use the one, or some combination, that suits the patient's problem.
1. Contemplative, History-Oriented Response, also known as "CHOR."
2. Fast Action Saves Time pathway, also known as "FAST."

II. Information Processing During the Golden Minute

Three types of information "set the tone" for diagnosis, assessment, and treatment during the first 60 seconds. This information must be obtained quickly and efficiently. **Note:** often these facts can be gathered before arrival at the scene.

A. Clinical History

While the patient is being stabilized, the EMT should obtain relevant data, including past medical history, history of present symptoms, chief complaint, medications and recent changes in medication dosages. Important historical features include:

1. Mechanism of injury (in trauma cases). See Section IIB.
2. Is this a *new* problem or a worsening of an *old* problem? Let the patient be your guide! This is especially important in the following conditions:
   a. Congestive heart failure (CHF).
   b. Chronic obstructive pulmonary disease (COPD).
   c. Asthma: Has patient ever required intubation in the past? What medications seem to work for patient? How long has this attack lasted?
   d. Altered mental status: Recent or preexisting? Associated fever?
   e. Medication reactions: Ask patient whether there is the possibility of adverse reaction. Has medication dose changed recently?
   f. Respiratory distress. Immediately consider the following:
      i. Pulmonary edema.
      ii. COPD.
      iii. Asthma.
      iv. Pneumonia.
      v. Allergic reaction.
      vi. Tension pneumothorax.
      vii. Foreign body aspiration.
   g. Seizures. Determine whether patient has a seizure disorder.

B. Mechanism of Injury

1. Critical information for multiple trauma victims:
   a. Was the victim in a high-speed or a low-speed motor vehicle accident?

b. In cases of violation of the passenger compartment: was the patient restrained or unrestrained (passive restraints such as deployed airbag; seat belt; child safety seat)?
c. Was the victim thrown from a vehicle?
d. Was the mechanism of injury blunt or penetrating?
e. With lacerations, injury to tendons and nerves is likely.
f. Is the neck hyperextended?
g. How far did the victim fall? (A fall from a height of three stories or greater has 50% mortality.)

C. **Evidence at the Emergency Scene**
  1. Critical information to guide the EMT during Golden-Minute assessment of **major trauma**:
     a. Blood loss: A large amount of blood at the scene suggests severe hemorrhage, but absence of blood does not rule out severe blood loss.
     b. Level of consciousness: Any alteration or depression of consciousness in a setting of major trauma is indication for rapid stabilization and transport.
     c. Distance from vehicle: Victims thrown from a vehicle are likely to have severe internal injuries with hemorrhage.
     d. Vital signs. Use initial vital signs as a guide to rapid intervention. Respiratory rate greater than 30, heart rate greater than 110, and systolic blood pressure (BP) less than 100 indicate necessity for immediate stabilization. **Note:** Drop in BP is a late sign of shock.
  2. Critical information to guide the EMT during Golden Minute assessment of **medical emergencies**:
     a. In cases of cardiopulmonary arrest, was bystander CPR initiated? If so, how long after the collapse?
     b. Have ABCs (airway, breathing, circulation) been maintained?
     c. Look for evidence of toxic ingestion or drug overdose:
        i. Seizures in the setting of cardiac arrest suggest a possible "upper" overdose (cocaine, tricyclics, etc.).
        ii. Severe respiratory depression suggests a "downer" (heroin, tranquilizers, etc.) overdose.
     d. Is CPR in progress? If so, prognosis is improved.

e. Check Medic-Alert bracelets, tags, necklaces (diabetes? anticoagulants? pacemaker?).

     f. Coma protocol. Administer 50 ccs D50W, 2.0 mg Narcan, and 100 mg thiamine IM if patient is comatose.

     g. General environmental condition. Evaluate the patient for the possibility of hypothermia or hyperthermia.

     h. Evaluate the home environment. Look for signs of a patient's inability to care for himself, drugs, alcohol, evidence of recent meals, medications.

III. Action Pathways for the Golden Minute
Fast Action Saves Time (FAST) vs. Contemplative, History-Oriented Response (CHOR) pathway

  A. **FAST** track is used whenever immediate intervention is necessary regardless of the clinical history. The following situations will require the FAST track:

     1. Cardiopulmonary respiratory arrest.
     2. Major trauma.
     3. Respiratory distress.
     4. Apnea.
     5. Severe CHF.
     6. Drug overdose.
     7. Coma.
     8. Severe asthma.
     9. Seizures.
    10. Shock.
    11. "C-spine" injury.
    12. Infant distress.
    13. Child abuse.

  B. The **CHOR** track is used in non–life-threatening situations; in these cases the most accurate course of action is determined primarily by historical features of the illness. This approach is recommended in the following:

     1. Geriatric patients with altered mental status, fever, falls, adverse drug reactions, syncope, or gradual deterioration.

     2. Patients with chest pain who are not hemodynamically unstable.

3. Patients with shortness of breath who do not appear to have life-threatening respiratory distress.
4. Patients with syncope who are hemodynamically stable and who do not have cardiac arrhythmias.

IV. Golden Minute Assessment for the 60-Second EMT

A. **The Golden Minute Evaluation.**
Choosing and implementing appropriate treatment protocols requires that the EMT reach the correct diagnosis as soon as possible. The Golden Minute exam includes evaluation of ABCs: airway, breathing, cardiovascular and hemodynamic status, neurologic status and severe fractures of distal extremities. Within the time frame of the Golden Minute, **the patient's vital signs must be maintained regardless of the underlying cause of the patient's deterioration.**

B. **The Golden Minute Nine-point Plan in Multiple Trauma**
1. **Vital Signs:** Obtain the vital signs immediately as a guide to aggressiveness of therapy and to provide important **diagnostic data.** Establish and maintain the patient's airway; intubate patient with respiratory distress if in doubt. Place large-bore IV lines when hypotension is present. Treat life-threatening arrhythmias.
2. **Primary Survey:**
    a. Airway, **C**-spine control, **B**reathing, and **C**irculation.
    b. Treat coma with standard three-drug protocol.
    c. Control external hemorrhage sites and maintain vital signs with LR or NS.
    d. Monitor neurologic status with Glasgow Coma Scale.
    e. Adequately expose patient for accurate physical assessment.
3. **Secondary Survey:** Search for other sources of blood loss.
4. **Circulation Management:**
    a. Apply direct pressure to bleeding sites.
    b. Place pneumatic antishock garment (PASG) if there is subdiaphragmatic hemorrhagic shock or unstable pelvis.
    c. Be aggressive with IV lines and fluid administration. Limit initial resuscitation to 2000 ml unless physician-directed.

5. **Cardiac Monitor:**
   a. Treat life-threatening arrhythmias.
   b. Make sure that hypovolemia is corrected before vasopressor agents are used.
6. **Fracture stabilization.**
7. **Neurovascular status assessment.**
8. **Tension Pneumothorax:** Consider the possibility of tension pneumothorax in a patient with respiratory distress who does not respond to stabilization procedures.
9. **Teamwork.**

V. The Golden Minute Curriculum for the 60-Second EMT
A. **The Search** for the 60-Second EMT
B. **Medical Emergencies**
   1. The 60-Second Assessment of Syncope.
   2. The 60-Second Assessment of Chest Pain.
   3. The 60-Second Assessment of Cardiac Arrest.
   4. The 60-Second Abdominal Assessment.
   5. The 60-Second Assessment of the HIV Patient.
   6. The 60-Second Coma Assessment.
   7. The 60-Second Toxicology Assessment.
   8. The 60-Second HazMat Assessment.
   9. The 60 Second Respiratory Exam.
   10. The 60 Second Assessment of Thermoregulatory Disorders.
   11. The 60 Second Neurologic Assessment.
   12. The 60 Second Geriatric Assessment.
   13. The 60-Second Pediatric Assessment.

C. **Traumatic Emergencies**
The 60-Second Assessment of Multiple Trauma.

D. **Communication Emergencies**
The 60-Second Case Presentation.

VI. CONCLUSION
The Golden Minute evaluation can be the key to rapid treatment and assessment. The evaluation requires assessing multiple organ systems simultaneously and keeping a mental log of many factors.

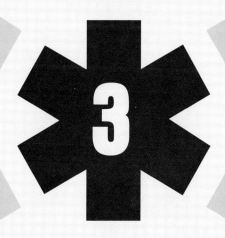

The 60-Second
Syncope Assessment

Tim Scott and I arranged to meet at the base station hospital. He told me to look for a sign that read "Paramedic Review Course—The 60-Second EMT." I had no trouble finding it. I arrived early and snuck into the lecture hall through a back door. I tiptoed down the stairs quietly and took a seat in the back of the room so that I would not interrupt the class. Tim was finishing a lecture to a group of EMTs. The place was packed. Everyone's eyes were focused intently on him; some students even looked a little tense. I realized why. The EMTs in this audience would soon be taking their paramedic certification exams. A round of applause greeted the end of Scott's session. As the students filed out, I made my way down to the podium.

A number of people had told me about Tim Scott. One of the finest EMTs in the state, he was almost as much a legend as Jerry Donnelly. I had heard from a reliable source that Scott was just the man to tell me what Donnelly had done to earn his reputation as the 60-Second EMT. From all accounts, the two had worked very closely together: first, in the field and then, later, developing prehospital protocols for the county's EMS system. In the process, Scott himself had become one of the most active disseminators of the 60-second program.

"So you're the one that wants to know all about Jerry Donnelly," Scott said as I stepped up to the podium.

"Not exactly," I said sheepishly.

I had already learned that no single person could tell me everything there was to know about Jerry Donnelly. Scott started to erase the blackboard. I had the feeling that he was preparing to give another lecture. For a moment, I thought maybe he had misunderstood the purpose of our get-together.

> Thorough primary and secondary surveys are a top priority for all EMTs.

"What I'm really interested in knowing, Tim," I continued, "is why Donnelly is called the 60-Second EMT. Apparently, the guy can assess patients faster than the speed of light. Fact or fiction?"

"Donnelly's fast. No doubt about that," admitted Scott. "But he never uses his speed and quick wits at the expense of a thorough primary and secondary survey. These components of patient assessment are a top priority for all EMTs, and Jerry is no exception. In his 60-second system for EMTs, there's no neglecting the ABCs. Standards are standards and he'll be the first to say so."

"But his 60-second approach goes beyond standards and protocols, doesn't it?" I asked.

"Sure it does. That's what makes The 60-Second EMT so unique," Scott assured me. "You see, Jerry's discipline and adherence to protocols may be enough to make him solid and competent in his profession. But his talents and skills in the prehospital setting transcend competence. They're in a league of their own. Everyone knows Jerry has a special quality. A kind of curiosity, you might call it—a desire to probe deeply into a case and get to its bottom. He's a real detective when it comes to getting a history and sifting out the details of a particular case."

> Syncopal episodes are among the most difficult cases an EMT sees because he has to decide quickly whether the patient's underlying event is life-threatening or not.

"Sounds like the guy's some sleuth out in the field," I said. "Can you give me some examples?"

"Sure. There is one kind of prehospital encounter in which Donnelly is an absolute master," Scott confided. "I'm talking about his uncanny ability to assess and manage patients with syncope."

"Those are some of the more challenging cases EMTs and paramedics see," I offered.

"You bet they are," he said. "And some of the sickest. Fortunately, the 60-Second Syncope Assessment is very useful for splitting diagnostic hairs in these situations. Jerry's 60-second program can teach the EMT to become extraordinarily skilled at dividing syncopal patients into two groups: first, urgent, life-threatening syncope caused by cardiac, hemorrhagic, and neurologic events and, second, nonurgent syncope caused by vasovagal (vasodepressor) and other forms of syncope, for example, tussive syncope, micturition syncope, and stress-induced syncope."

Making this distinction in the prehospital setting is the key to rational management of syncopal patients in the field. I was excited that Donnelly had actually incorporated this feature into his 60-second equation.

Scott picked up a piece of chalk and wrote, "Dizziness and Syncope" on the blackboard. Then he turned around, took a deep breath, and lit up with a smile. I settled in for what turned out to be the most illuminating lecture on syncope I had ever heard.

"EMTs get plenty of calls to see patients who have had a syncopal episode," Scott began. "They're among the most difficult cases an EMT sees because he has to decide quickly whether the patient's underlying event is life-threatening or not. Frequently, the precipitating event is already over by the time the EMT arrives, and additional clues are hard to come by."

I had been in that predicament many times. "You're working with a blank slate in these cases," I added.

"You're right. But sometimes, it's even worse than that," Scott explained. "You may not even know there's been a syncopal event. In other words, the syncopal episode may not even be the presenting complaint."

In all cases of unexplained trauma, syncope should be considered as a possible diagnosis.

Scott went on. "In these cases, the EMT may have to work backwards to determine whether an unwitnessed syncopal episode is actually the underlying cause of a traumatic event such as, let's say, a head injury sustained in a car accident or a broken hip resulting from a fall. There may be some real sleuthing involved. Syncope can be a very elusive diagnosis."

"What can the 60-Second EMT do about this problem?" I asked. "What's special about Donnelly's approach in these situations?"

"Well, the first point," continued Scott, "is not to miss a case of syncope. Donnelly's 60-second approach stresses that in all cases of unexplained trauma, especially in the geriatric group, syncope should be considered as a possible diagnosis. Whenever an elderly person falls and breaks his hip or sustains some other significant injury, the EMT has to entertain the possibility that a syncopal episode is the underlying event. The same index of suspicion applies to single-car motor vehicle accidents. Again, a blackout spell or seizure may have been the precipitating event. If the patient is alert and talking, the EMT can usually obtain this history within the first minute of the encounter."

Scott argued convincingly that many cases involving syncope have "snakes hidden in the grass." He also emphasized that Donnelly's 60-second assessment offered a comprehensive scheme for detecting these patients early in the prehospital setting. Naturally I was interested in getting more specific information, so I sat back and listened.

"Jerry treats the patient with syncope much as he would someone having a myocardial infarction: with a sense of urgency," continued Scott. "When treating these patients, he's always prepared for the worst-case scenario. The 60-Second EMT is taught to think

Causes of Syncope and Dizziness

1. Vasodepressor syncope
2. Seizure
3. Orthostatic syncope
   a. Hypovolemia or adrenal insufficiency
   b. Prolonged recumbency
   c. Physical deconditioning
   d. Venous insufficiency
   e. Peripheral neuropathies or drugs
   f. Autonomic insufficiency
   g. Micturition syncope
4. Cardiac syncope
   a. Morgagni-Adams-Stokes syndromes
   b. Bradyarrhythmias
   c. Tachyarrhythmias
   d. Sick sinus syndrome
   e. Aortic stenosis
   f. Idiopathic hypertrophic subaortic stenosis
   g. Massive myocardial infarction
   h. Pulmonary embolism
   i. Atrial myxoma
   j. Carotid sinus syncope
5. Cerebrovascular causes
   a. Drop attacks and akinetic fainting spells
   b. Atherosclerosis
6. Hypoglycemia
7. Narcolepsy
8. Hyperventilation
9. Vertigo

of the most ominous possibilities first. For example, a bona fide syncopal episode can be caused by heart block, hemorrhage, respiratory distress, life-threatening arrhythmia, seizures, and many other conditions."

"But how does the EMT prepare for these contingencies?" I inquired. "And how does he evaluate the seriousness of a syncopal event?" Those were questions I had never had answered to my satisfaction.

"I'm glad you asked, because that's a key part of the 60-second exam in these patients," Scott bounced back with enthusiasm.

The 60-Second EMT is taught to think of the most ominous possibilities first.

"If the patient seems in the least bit unstable—if there is any suggestion of a serious underlying event, cardiac or hemodynamic—Jerry will go right to work with the O_2, cardiac monitor, and IV line."

Scott began writing a list of conditions that cause syncope on the blackboard: (1) Ventricular arrhythmias, (2) Supraventricular tachycardia, (3) Seizures, (4) Orthostatic hypotension, (5) Gastrointestinal bleeding (6) Medication reaction, (7) Drug-induced orthostatic hypotension. . . .

"But the list of problems that cause syncope is too long," I countered. "How can the paramedic or EMT possibly get a handle on what's going on within the first minute?"

"That never intimidates Jerry. And it won't be any problem for you once you get the hang of the 60-Second Syncope Exam."

I only wished that his prediction would come true. Nevertheless, he was very convincing.

"Let me tell you about a case and I think you'll get the idea," Scott said. "Last month, Jerry and I were called out to see an elderly hotel clerk who had passed out while sitting in a chair at the reception desk of a hotel lobby. Upon arriving, we were led to a man in his 70s who was lying on the carpet and surrounded by a circle of well-dressed tourists. We noted a blood pressure of 120/70, and the cardiac monitor revealed a sinus tachycardia at a rate of 110. His respirations were regular and SaO_2 was 90% on room air. We put an IV line in as a precaution and started the patient on O_2 by nasal cannula. That was Jerry's idea. The man's mental status rapidly cleared a few moments after we arrived, so Jerry asked him some questions about what had happened."

I was very interested in hearing Donnelly's line of questioning. I knew that I might discover the substance of his 60-second secrets in Jerry's interview of the patient, which Scott described.

" 'Where were you sitting when things went black?' Jerry inquired.

" 'In the chair there,' the man answered in a frail voice.

" 'Are you on any medications?' Jerry asked lickety-split.

" 'No,' the man answered.

" 'Do you have any history of heart disease?'

" 'No.'

" 'Do you have a seizure disorder?' probed Jerry.

" 'No.'

" 'Do you have an irregular heartbeat, or any history of extra beats, or problems with your heart rhythm?'

" 'Can't say that I do,' the man said, and then added, 'You know, I really think I'm ok now. You boys can run along. I don't think I need to go to the hospital. Thanks for all your help.' "

"I guess it only took Donnelly a minute to figure out that there was probably nothing wrong," I supposed.

"Maybe you should reserve judgment for now," Scott suggested. "Some EMTs might have followed the old man's advice and left, but not Jerry. His stubbornness in these situations can be one of his greatest assets." Scott continued the story. "He took the patient's pulse again, turned to me, and said, 'You know, Tim, this guy has a resting heart rate of 110 when he's lying here quietly on the floor. It's too fast. And his skin feels a little clammy. We'd better take him to the hospital.' ''

" 'What do you think is going on, Jerry?' I asked. 'He's got a regular heart rate and his blood pressure is normal,' I pointed out.

" 'Maybe his pressure is normal, but maybe it isn't,' I remember Jerry insisting, as he quickly considered a more ominous explanation. Then, in a stroke of brilliance, he said, 'For a man of his age, a pressure of 120/70 might actually be low. In fact, I bet his normal pressure is higher than that; this guy is probably hypotensive and hypovolemic.' ''

"So what did Donnelly do?"

"He took orthostatic pulses and blood pressures, and sure enough the man had a 15-point systolic drop and a 30 beat per minute–increase in his heart rate."

This analysis gave me a glimpse into the inner workings of Donnelly's "60-second" mind.

Scott continued. "You have to admit that this point was well taken. So, almost instinctively, Jerry repeated his secondary survey and discovered that the man's pants were soaked through at the crotch. 'Look, Tim,' he said, pointing to the wet area. This guy had urinary incontinence when he had his syncopal episode. That does it. Let's open up that IV and get him to the hospital.' ''

"Well, was Donnelly right?" I asked somewhat excitedly.

"The man's condition remained stable with O_2 during transport," continued Scott. "Then, on the way to the base station, Jerry asked the key question. 'Have you had any change in your bowel movements lately? Any dark, tarry stools?'

" 'Now that you mention it, my bowel movements have been very black during the past few days,' the old man recalled. By the time we rolled through the emergency department doors Jerry had concluded that his patient had had a GI bleed, become hypotensive, and had a syncopal episode.

"The emergency department physician confirmed Donnelly's suspicion and his assessment of the victim's problem. The urinary incontinence, relatively low blood pressure, and resting sinus tachycardia had tipped Donnelly off to the seriousness of this man's blackout. This encounter was just one of many examples in which Donnelly used his 60-second approach to uncover a problem."

Scott replaced the piece of chalk and sat down at a desk next to mine. I could see that it made him happy just to be talking about

Donnelly's approach to the syncopal patient. It was obvious that Donnelly had really inspired him.

"What's unique about Jerry," Scott commented, "is his ability to ask questions that are precise enough to differentiate between urgent and less urgent causes of syncope and dizziness."

"Can you be more specific?" I asked.

"No problem," Scott answered. "Jerry's 60-second assessment of the syncopal patient is a powerful yet practical clinical tool that's simple enough for every EMT to remember and use."

"Where does he start?" I asked.

"Well, that depends on how stable the patient is. If the syncopal episode is over and the patient is relatively stable and alert, Donnelly first asks the patient to define his or her syncopal episode in precise detail. He wants to know if things actually went black, or if he or she just had some dizziness. A bona fide syncopal episode has occurred if the patient has completely lost consciousness. He or she has to have actually blacked out. Characterizing the exact nature of the blackout from the outset, and distinguishing syncope from a presyncopal attack—the feeling of almost blacking out—or vertigo is a top priority.

"And if the patient can't give an accurate history, which is often the case, Donnelly asks bystanders, family members, or other witnesses. Frequently, they can paint the most accurate picture of what actually happened."

"Once Donnelly determines that a syncopal episode has occurred, where does he go from there?" I asked.

"If he's confident that there has been a real syncopal episode, Jerry will delve into the situational variables. He asks whether the episode occurred in a warm, crowded room and if the patient was standing when he passed out. He asks if alcohol was involved. He knows this combination is a setup for vasovagal syncope, in which the heart rate slows dramatically, leading to decreased cerebral perfusion and, eventually, a syncopal attack."

I liked this approach. It seemed very straightforward. I wanted to know more.

"What's the importance of distinguishing vasovagal syncope from other types of blackouts?" I asked.

"Vasovagal syncope can—and usually does—occur in people who do not have serious underlying disease," explained Scott.

If the patient can't give an accurate history, ask bystanders, family members, or other witnesses.

Causes of Vasovagal Syncope

1. Emotional distress
2. Prolonged standing in warm, crowded rooms
3. Pain
4. Prolonged bed rest or fasting
5. Mild blood loss
6. Anemia
7. Fever

"More often than not, people who have had a vasovagal attack lose consciousness only momentarily and recover very quickly once they're in the supine position. It's uncommon for vasovagal syncope to result in significant traumatic injury, and rarely is there associated incontinence. These are the kinds of things that have to go through the mind of the 60-Second EMT."

> Vasovagal syncope can occur in people who do not have serious underlying disease.

I was pleased that Scott was willing to share Donnelly's clinical pearls. This is what I had come to hear.

"But that's not all," stressed Scott. "Within the first minute of his prehospital encounter with a syncopal patient, Donnelly also determines what position the patient was in when the syncopal episode occurred. That's key. If it occurred with the individual in the supine or sitting position, Donnelly is immediately alerted to the possibility of a cardiac event, such as complete heart block or, perhaps, a life-threatening arrhythmia. Of course, syncope in the supine position is especially worrisome."

"Let me see if I'm following you here," I said. "You mean Donnelly reasons that orthostatic and vasovagal syncope are usually position-dependent and, therefore, rarely occur when a person is in the supine or sitting position. I suppose that means you have to consider an arrhythmia, heart block, or a neurologic ischemic event if the syncopal event occurs while the patient is sitting or supine."

> If there are any associated chest pain, shortness of breath, recent fainting spells, or palpitations take cardiac precautions immediately.

"That's right," Tim coached. "So what conclusion can you draw from this?"

I thought for a moment, then said, "I guess that means that the 60-Second EMT should consider a more ominous cause for syncope if it occurs when the patient is in a supine or sitting position."

"That's exactly the point!" Tim replied. "And, to fine-tune his diagnosis even further, Jerry asks the syncopal victim if there was any associated chest pain, shortness of breath, recent fainting spells, or palpitations. If he answers affirmatively to any of these questions, Jerry takes cardiac precautions immediately. You see, the 60-Second EMT can glean this information within the first minute of the patient encounter. That's what's so beautiful about Donnelly's approach. It's tailor-made for the symptom he's analyzing and, therefore, saves an incredible amount of time."

I was impressed with this scheme. It was fast and direct.

"It's extraordinary to see him analyze these factors right on the spot. By the way, have you seen him work in the field?" Scott inquired.

"No, I haven't had the pleasure," I replied.

Scott went on like a proud student who had learned his lessons well.

"Donnelly makes the point that if there is no warning before a syncopal episode, then a cardiac event, orthostatic syncope, or a seizure is much more probable than a vasovagal episode. In such a case, he's quick to put the monitor on and look for rhythm abnormalities. And one more thing: if there is significant trauma—a fracture, large hematoma, or laceration—accompanying the blackout, Jerry's index of suspicion for a serious cardiac arrhythmia, hemorrhage, or seizure is significantly increased. He considers trauma in the setting of syncope a sign of urgency that demands precautionary measures."

If there is no warning before a syncopal episode, then a cardiac event, orthostatic syncope, or a seizure is much more probable than a vasovagal episode.

"Are there any other clues he relies on to draw these kinds of conclusions?" I wondered.

"Sure," Scott rebounded. "Jerry also looks for tongue-biting or shoulder dislocation, which might suggest that a syncopal attack was caused by a seizure. If there has been urinary or fecal incontinence, he knows within the first minute of his contact with the victim that the syncopal attack needs to be taken seriously—very seriously—because incontinence suggests a non-vasovagal cause of the syncopal episode. As I just mentioned, these usually fall into serious, life-threatening categories. If bystanders have noted cyanosis, respiratory stridor, or apnea, Donnelly suspects life-threatening respiratory or cardiac etiologies and acts accordingly."

"What do you mean by 'accordingly'?" I asked.

"The 60-Second Syncope Assessment demands an aggressive

approach to patients who show signs of respiratory, neurologic, or hemodynamic compromise during, before, or after their period of unconsciousness," Tim explained. "In these situations, the 60-Second EMT starts an IV and cardiac monitor, draws blood samples, administers O_2 as needed, and, if there are signs of hypovolemia, administers volume expander. If the patient is still unconscious, he institutes the coma protocol."

Donnelly's 60-second approach to the patient with syncope seemed solid. It was systematic, rational, and relied on key historical features to orient the EMT. Within the first minute or so, Donnelly evaluated the urgency of the situation on the basis of specific situational and physical variables. Then, if the data warranted it, he instituted the FAST track of supportive management.

"Any other key aspects of the 60-second exam in the syncopal patient?" I asked.

"Absolutely," Scott replied. "The longer the duration of the syncopal episode, the more Jerry worries. And with good reason. Victims of vasovagal attacks are usually unconscious for only a matter of seconds. But patients with heart block, serious arrhythmias, and seizures can be unconscious for a few minutes, or even longer, before regaining consciousness."

"What about the recovery phase?" I inquired.

"How quickly syncopal patients regain consciousness is another important part of Donnelly's 60-second equation," confirmed Scott. "Jerry emphasizes that patients with vasovagal syncope usually recover consciousness quite rapidly once they are supine and the inciting event is over."

"And what about other causes of syncope?" I asked.

Scott explained. "Patients who 'black out' from seizures or other neurologic conditions generally have a longer recovery period—a prolonged postictal phase—before regaining lucidity. The same is true of patients who've had catastrophic intracerebral or subarachnoid hemorrhages, or long periods of cerebral anoxia from a cardiac arrhythmia or full arrest. They may never regain consciousness in the field."

Scott's explanation of how to distinguish urgent from non-urgent causes of syncope was impeccable. But I wanted to know more about the 60-second approach to patients who had syncope because of adverse drug reactions. This point is so important, especially in the elderly population.

"How can the 60-Second Syncope Assessment help me with patients who might have had a drug reaction?" I inquired.

"I'm glad you asked, because there are many questions Donnelly asks to assess the role drugs play in a syncopal episode," explained Scott while writing on the blackboard. "If the victim is conscious, Donnelly obtains a very quick medication history. He asks first about drugs that can cause orthostatic syncope, such as diuretics, beta-blockers, and antihypertensives. Then he asks about narcotic analgesics, anticholinergic drugs such as tricyclic antidepressants, tranquilizers, and phenothiazines. Finally, he inquires about cardiac drugs such as quinidine, Norpace®, and digoxin since they not only can cause hypotension, but can also cause the arrhythmias they are supposed to prevent. These are the most likely offenders.

> **Obtain a very quick medication history.**

"Of course, he's always sure to ask whether there's a history of diabetes or insulin use. We've seen cases in which hypoglycemia caused someone to have a syncopal episode. I've seen Donnelly pinpoint the cause of syncopal attacks right on the spot with this kind of probing. Weaving together the story of a syncopal event usually doesn't take him very long. He can amass a lot of information in less than a minute. That's because he knows exactly what his line of questioning is going to be. The guy is so well rehearsed, he could act in a Broadway play. There's never a moment's hesitation, and every line is right on cue."

"Doesn't that distract him from the job of supporting the patient's vital signs and attending to the ABCs?" I inquired.

"No way! While Jerry is getting this information together, he's hooking the patient up to a monitor and looking for signs of heart block and arrhythmias. If he detects a supraventricular tachycardia—let's say, atrial fibrillation with a rapid ventricular response, bigeminy, ventricular tachycardia, or multifocal PVCs—he institutes treatment protocols for cardiac arrhythmias."

> **Never take chances with people who have a syncopal episode and chest pain.**

"And what if the victim reports chest pain along with the syncopal episode?" I asked.

"The 60-Second EMT knows that's a red flag if there ever was one," Scott answered. "Jerry never takes chances with people who have a syncopal episode and chest pain. I've seen him save lives because of his vigilance with this high-risk group. He knows these two symptoms are a lethal combination. They frequently indicate that the patient has had cardiac syncope from an arrhythmia caused by a myocardial infarction.

"Donnelly looks at it this way," Scott continued. "The 60-Second EMT approaches this symptom with the understanding that there are both life-threatening and non–life-threatening causes for syncope and dizziness. As a rule, vasovagal attacks are the least worrisome. And the most common. On the other hand, cardiac syncope, orthostatic syncope, medication-induced syncope, and syncope caused by volume depletion, hemorrhage, and seizures require immediate action and transport. Using the 60-Second Syncope Assessment, the EMT can make this differentiation with a relative degree of accuracy in a minimum amount of time. Go out and see how Jerry does it yourself. That'll convince you."

I did not need to. I was already convinced. I had just learned some invaluable pearls. After Scott finished Donnelly's 60-Second Syncope Exam, I felt that I had found what I was looking for.

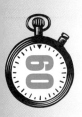

SYNCOPE

There are certain *"red flags"* that Donnelly uses to quickly suspect dangerous causes of syncope requiring ALS treatment and transport. When any of these is present, the EMT must consider the cause of the syncope to be either cardiac or neurologic. If all red flags are absent, the patient will probably only need BLS services.

The "ESP" approach to syncope divides assessment into three distinct phases: Early premonitory phase, Syncopal phase, and Post–syncopal phase, each having its own red flags.

Early, premonitory phase red flags: Stay on the "SCENT" of the problem:

- **S**upine posture when syncope occurs
- **C**ardiac symptoms just before syncope (chest pains, shortness of breath, palpitations)
- **E**lderly patients who should always be considered to have a serious cause of their syncope
- **N**o warning of the syncope, which should always imply cardiac or neurologic cause
- **T**rauma associated with the syncope (either as a result or cause)

Syncopal phase red flags: During the syncope (period of unconsciousness), watch for the following "TIPS":

- **T**ongue-biting
- **I**ncontinence of urine or, especially, of stool
- **P**rolonged duration of unconsciousness
- **S**eizure activity

Post–syncopal phase red flags: Watch for these like Charley "CHAN":

- **C**onfusion
- **H**eadaches
- **A**bnormal vital signs
- **N**eurological dysfunction (especially *focal* dysfunction)

4

The 60-Second Assessment of Chest Pain

ot only was Bill Hawkins an EMT, he was Jerry Donnelly's regular running partner. The two had run in a number of major races together including the Boston Marathon and the Cascade Runoff in Portland, Oregon. Not surprisingly, perhaps, Bill's area of specialty was heart disease. He was an AHA-ACLS instructor and had helped to introduce several new cardiac drugs into the prehospital protocols. Hawkins' interest in exercise physiology and cardiac disorders had made him an invaluable consultant to Donnelly's 60-Second EMT program. I knew he would be a gold mine of information.

I met Hawkins at an outdoor track near the medical school. It was a clear, crisp autumn day. I could see Hawkins' yellow and black running shorts bobbing up and down in the distance. Including fire-engine-red Reeboks, his outfit was brighter than the leaves that had fallen onto the asphalt track. He saw me waiting for him in the bleachers as he circled and indicated with a flash of his index finger that he had one more lap to go. I watched him build up speed for the last lap and then shift into high gear down the homestretch. The guy was a human piston. Just looking at him was enough to give me chest pain.

He jogged to a stop about 100 yards in front of me. I went out to greet him. By the time we were face to face, Bill was barely panting. I could hardly believe it. I remember thinking that his coronary arteries were probably as clean as a whistle.

"Sorry you had to wait," Hawkins said. "I'm building up for a ten-mile run next month, so I've got to get my five miles in today."

"No problem," I answered. I could make out every muscle in his calves and thighs. We walked over to the bleachers and sat down.

"I talked to Jerry yesterday," continued Hawkins as he untied his running shoes and took off his sweatshirt. "He said you might be calling me. When I asked him how he knew about our meeting, he was kind of elusive about the whole thing."

"Maybe I should explain. . . ."

"There's no need to," Hawkins interrupted. "Everyone wants to know about Jerry Donnelly's 60-Second EMT Program. It's made the guy a legend around these parts. I put two and two together and figured he was sending you to ask me about the 60-Second Chest Pain Exam. So, tell me, am I right?"

"As a matter of fact, you are," I confessed.

"I don't know if Jerry told you or not," Hawkins continued, "but the 60-Second Chest Pain Assessment was the first module we developed for The 60-Second EMT."

"No, he didn't." I was surprised. "Why do you think Donnelly chose chest pain to spearhead the 60-Second EMT Program?"

"Because chest pain is one of the most common problems EMTs encounter in the prehospital environment," Hawkins answered. "It can be the presenting symptom of several diseases, some of them life-threatening."

> Chest pain is one of the most common problems EMTs encounter in the prehospital environment.

I thought for a moment about this and then added, "It's true. You have to work fast in patients with chest pain. In some cases, 60 seconds is about all the time you have to begin some very critical procedures. You may have to regulate an arrhythmia, relieve chest pain, or treat congestive heart failure."

"That's right," agreed Hawkins. "Jerry developed this 60-second exam so EMTs could distinguish, early in their assessment, between conditions such as myocardial infarction, which are extremely urgent and require aggressive therapy, and others such as pneumonia, pleurisy, and anxiety reactions, which are less urgent. Jerry thought if he could develop a 60-second assessment that would help EMTs discriminate among causes of chest pain, he'd really be on to something."

"Well, do you think he was?" I inquired.

"No doubt about it," said the runner. "In fact, I was with Jerry the first time he took his 60-Second Chest Pain Assessment for a 'test run' in the field."

"I'd like to hear about that," I answered, sensing that Bill's account would shed new light on my investigation.

"It was a hot summer day, and Jerry and I were riding together," Bill began. "The base station dispatcher called and told us we had a 76-year-old man with chest pain waiting for us at the yacht club. The report indicated that he was diaphoretic and looked pretty bad. We made a beeline for the place, Code 3."

"How did the 60-Second Exam help you in this situation?" I asked. "Sounds like the guy was having an MI."

"Well, that's the kind of mind-set I had, too," Hawkins remembered. "But as we were en route, I realized I'd gotten a little lazy in my thinking about chest pain."

"What gave you that feeling?" I inquired.

"Well, to tell you the truth," he confided, "it was Jerry. He made me feel a little insecure about the way I approached chest pain. He started rattling off key points in the 60-Second Chest Pain Assessment. And before we reached the sick man, I had a whole new perspective on chest pain as a presenting complaint."

"In what sense?" I queried.

"In the sense that chest pain can be caused by several disease processes, and if the EMT knows the symptoms and signs of each, he or she can arrive at an accurate assessment within the first minute of the prehospital encounter."

"You really think that's possible?" I asked with astonishment.

"Yes, I do. If you ask the right questions and know how to interpret irregularities in the patient's vital signs, you can rapidly narrow down the possible causes of chest pain," he explained. "But there is an art to it."

> **If you ask the right questions and know how to interpret irregularities in the patient's vital signs, you can rapidly narrow down the possible causes of chest pain.**

"Sounds like the 60-Second Chest Pain Exam is powerful stuff," I commented.

"It is," said the runner. "And just how powerful became clear to me as we cruised down the highway. Jerry asked me if I'd ever heard of the 'CRAMPS' mnemonic for chest pain. I said no."

"CRAMPS?" I asked, to be sure I'd gotten it right.

"Jerry said that every EMT and paramedic should know how to use the CRAMPS mnemonic for chest pain. The letters stand for Costochondral chest wall pain, Rebound pain from withdrawal of

---

The CRAMPS Mnemonic for Chest Pain

Costochondral chest wall pain
Rebound pain from withdrawal of cardiac medications
Angina
   Aortic aneurysm
   Anxiety
Myocardial infarction
Pneumonia
   Pericarditis
   Pneumothorax
   Pulmonary embolism
   Pleurisy
Spasm of the esophagus

cardiac medications, **A**ngina, **A**ortic aneurysm, **A**nxiety, **M**yocardial infarction, **P**neumonia, **P**ericarditis, **P**neumothorax, **P**ulmonary embolism, **P**leurisy, and **S**pasm of the esophagus."

"Hmmm, CRAMPS. . . ." I thought about it for a few seconds. "It really does cover all the important causes of chest pain, doesn't it?" I said.

"It surely does," agreed Hawkins. "Anyway, let me finish telling you about the patient. We arrived at the yacht club and found an elderly man complaining of severe chest pain; he was diaphoretic and short of breath. It looked to me as if the guy was having an MI, so I hooked him up to the cardiac monitor, gave him moderate-flow O_2, and Jerry started asking questions based on the 60-Second EMT Plan. He explored all the possibilities. I could almost hear the word 'CRAMPS' clicking through his brain."

"The 60-Second EMT in action?" I inquired.

"You wouldn't believe it!" Hawkins said. "First, Jerry recorded a blood pressure of 190/130 in the right arm. I didn't think much about that at first, but this value started Jerry along a specific line of questioning. He wanted to know if the patient had a history of high blood pressure. Which he did. He asked if the chest pain radiated to the back. The patient said 'Yes.' He asked if it was a constant pain. Again, the answer was affirmative. Then, Jerry asked him if it was relieved by nitroglycerin. The patient said he'd taken four nitros without any relief. Then he asked him if the pain radiated in the arms, neck, or jaw. The answer was 'No.' There was something about this patient's history that didn't exactly click with myocardial infarction. So Jerry unwrapped the cuff and took the blood pressure in his left arm. It was only 140/95, a significant deviation from the right arm."

"So what did Donnelly make of all this?" I asked.

"Well, the possibility of an MI was still high on the list. It had to be. But the radiation of the pain into the back, the hypertension, and the discrepancy in blood pressure from one arm to the other led Jerry to the diagnosis of a possible thoracic aortic aneurysm. We notified the hospital to alert the on-call surgeon and transported the patient immediately."

I was impressed with Donnelly's assessment of this situation. "What finally happened?"

"The patient's pain continued during transport despite more nitroglycerin and morphine, which the doctor at medical resource approved en route. Fortunately, his vital signs remained stable," Hawkins said. "Jerry asked for clearance to go directly to a Level

I trauma hospital. When we arrived, the emergency physician agreed with Jerry's on-the-spot assessment. He called a cardiovascular surgeon, who sent the patient for an aortic angiogram. It turned out he had an aneurysm.''

"Pretty impressive," I exclaimed.

"To say the least!" agreed the EMT. "When the emergency doctor found out Jerry's hunch was right, he walked up to him, shook his hand, and said, 'Good work . . . but Jerry, tell me, how on earth did you know it was an aneurysm?' ''

"Jerry just smiled and said, 'Did you ever hear of the 60-Second EMT?' ''

"What did the doctor say?" I asked.

"That he'd never heard of the 60-Second EMT. So Jerry took out his clean copy of the 60-Second Chest Pain Assessment and gave it to him.''

"The doctor marched right to the photocopy machine and made three copies of it. One for himself, one for the cardiac surgeon, and one for the resident. Can you believe it?" Hawkins enthused. "Anyway, that's how the 60-Second EMT was born.''

"And you really think the 60-Second Chest Pain Assessment helped Donnelly make the diagnosis of aortic aneurysm?" I inquired.

"I *know* it helped," Hawkins declared adamantly. "The 60-Second Chest Pain Exam stresses the importance of the patient's past and present history. It focuses on the duration and radiation of the pain pattern as well as associated symptoms. These are so important in differentiating urgent from nonurgent causes of chest pain.''

The 60-Second Chest Pain Exam focuses on the duration and radiation of the pain pattern as well as associated symptoms.

"But isn't it a little risky to jump to conclusions in the field about causes of chest pain?" I asked.

"Yes, in some respects it is, which is why Jerry always stresses one thing. Even if you think the patient isn't having an MI, chest pain in an older adult always needs to be treated with maximal precautions—cardiac monitor, nasal O_2, and frequent vital signs.''

"Can the 60-second approach improve on what paramedics already know about myocardial infarction?" I asked.

"Yes. In fact, it's especially valuable for assessing MI," Hawkins emphasized.

"Why?" I asked the marathoner.

Hawkins' explanation touched on something every EMT knows deep in his own heart (so to speak!).

"We have all learned that chest pain is the main symptom of myocardial infarction, but many of us don't go beyond that general concept," he said. "There is a tendency to get lazy and treat all chest pain alike. Sometimes we may forget to ask the kind of questions that really distinguish one cause of pain from another."

> The discomfort in myocardial in-farction is rarely a fleeting sensation.

"So how does the 60-second exam help?" I wanted to know.

"The 60-Second Chest Pain Assessment is useful because it helps the EMT paint a clear—and, in some respects, vivid—picture of what chest pain is like in patients with myocardial infarction and with other problems. It also stresses the ancillary symptoms associated with each."

This sounded like something worth knowing. "Can you be more specific?" I wanted details.

"Well, for one thing, the 60-Second Chest Pain Exam focuses on the duration, precise character, and radiation of the pain, and any associated findings."

"How long does the chest pain in myocardial infarction actually last?" I asked.

Hawkins clarified. "It can last on and off for hours, and sometimes there is a waxing and waning quality." He explained, "But the pain almost always lasts more than 20 minutes, and, usually, it continues for more like a half-hour or an hour. And it can last longer. It usually is not completely relieved by nitroglycerin. The key point is that the discomfort in myocardial infarction is rarely a fleeting sensation."

"How do patients describe the quality of the pain?" I inquired.

"They might describe it as a dull ache, a crushing pain, a pressure-like sensation, or a vise-like band across the chest. They might use the word tightness or tell you it feels like something heavy—would you believe an elephant?—is sitting on their chest," Hawkins explained. "Sometimes patients clench their fists tightly over the area of pain."

"What about sharp pain?" I asked.

"As a rule, the pain isn't sharp or stabbing; but it's almost always severe enough to stop patients in their tracks. If the pain forces the patients to stop whatever they are doing, you've got to put MI high on your list. And one more thing: patients in discomfort from the chest pain in myocardial infarction are typically very still. As a rule, it's not the kind of pain that causes writhing, although there are exceptions."

> If the pain forces the patients to stop whatever they are doing, you've got to put MI high on your list.

It did not take long for me to conclude that Donnelly's technique would enhance the way I approached patients with chest pain. There were many relevant questions that could be asked of patients within the first minute of prehospital encounter, and from what I had gathered thus far, Jerry Donnelly always had these on the tip of his tongue. After listening to Hawkins, I had to admit to myself that I really did not comprehend the important subtleties of this approach. The 60-Second Chest Pain Exam sounded as if it could be a real lifesaver.

"What other features in the patient's history can help clarify the origin of chest pain?" I asked.

Hawkins began some stretch exercises as he listed a number of key points. "Frequently, the chest pain in myocardial infarction is brought on by physical stress, emotional upset, a heavy meal, or extreme temperatures. And, of course, it's critical to ask about radiation of the pain."

"Why is that?" I queried.

"Because the pain of myocardial infarction radiates in a characteristic way," Hawkins explained. "Frequently, it just settles in the retrosternal area and produces a tight, heavy sensation or constant ache. And if the pain radiates down the left arm or into the neck or jaw, it strongly indicates pain of cardiac origin. And usually, the pain in myocardial infarction doesn't get worse with a deep breath like the discomfort in, let's say, pleurisy, pneumothorax, or pericarditis. These are important differential points."

> Frequently, the chest pain in MI is brought on by physical stress, emotional upset, a heavy meal, or extreme temperatures.

"You mean the chest pain in MI usually is not affected by breathing or positional variation?" I asked in an attempt to clarify Hawkins' point.

"That's right," he confirmed. "Let me give you an example. Once Jerry and I were called to see a middle-aged man with chest pain. He had had an upper respiratory infection for a few days; it was a flu-like illness, with lots of coughing. When we arrived, the guy was in excruciating pain. Initially, I thought he was having a myocardial infarction. He seemed to be in the right age group and had some risk factors such as smoking and mild obesity. So we took the necessary precautions."

"Was your hunch right?"

"Not in this case," Hawkins confessed. "But Jerry got to the heart of the matter in no time." Within the first minute or so," continued the marathoner, "he clarified the character of the discomfort. It turned out to be a very sharp, stabbing pain that increased at the end of every inspired breath. A pleuritic pain, in other words. In fact, if you studied the patient closely, you could see the guy was trying to minimize his breathing effort in an attempt to keep the pain at bay. You rarely see this in myocardial infarction. We transported the patient and it turned out he had an attack of pleurisy."

> Pleuritic pain is the inflammation of the two pleural layers covering the lung's surface.

"What causes pleuritic pain?" I asked.

"Inflammation of the two pleural layers covering the lung's surface. When the pleura are inflamed and patients take a deep breath, these two surfaces rub against each other and create pain. Sometimes the pain is very severe and the patient can barely sit still."

"Can you get pleuritic chest pain in other conditions?" I asked.

"Absolutely," Hawkins answered as he put his running shoes back on. "In fact, all the P's in 'CRAMPS' refer to conditions that can produce pleuritic pain."

"How convenient," I thought. " 'P' for Pleurisy, Pericarditis, Pneumonia, Pulmonary embolism, and Pneumothorax."

"Any condition that causes inflammation in the lung or heart can extend to the pleural surfaces of the lung and produce chest pain," elaborated Hawkins. "That's why chest pain in pneumonia is sometimes pleuritic in nature. The infection spreads to the covering of the lung. When this happens in pericarditis, the chest pain is frequently worse when the patient lies down."

> Any condition that causes inflammation in the lung or heart can extend to the pleural surfaces of the lung and produce chest pain.

"And when should the EMT consider a pneumothorax as a cause of chest pain?" I asked.

"That depends on whether the patient is old or young. In the younger age group, men with thin body frames who suddenly develop chest pain and shortness of breath are the most likely candidates for spontaneous pneumothorax. Among older patients, men and women with chronic lung disease, especially those with emphysema, are at risk. They can pop a bleb and collapse a lung. In most cases of spontaneous pneumothorax, however, breath sounds are diminished on one side and the EMT ought to pick this up in the primary survey."

The 60-Second Chest Exam seemed to offer a very discriminating assessment of chest pain. I pressed for more details.

"So it's really possible to confuse the chest pain of myocardial infarction with other conditions?" I queried.

"Yes, especially in the geriatric age group," answered Hawkins. "In pneumonia, chest pain may even be the patient's chief complaint. But in these cases, the presence of fever, a shaking chill, and increased sputum production ought to lead the EMT to this diagnosis. Elderly patients who are in nursing homes—especially if they've had a stroke—are at high risk for aspiration pneumonia. I'm sure you've seen cases in which chest discomfort was cited as their main symptom."

Indeed I had. In fact, I had always found it difficult to evaluate chest pain in the elderly, and from what I could gather, the 60-Second EMT addressed this problem well. Hawkins continued to divulge still more "pearls."

"The 60-Second EMT should determine from the outset whether or not there is any history of cardiac disease. This means finding out whether the patient has had angina, a previous infarction, or coronary artery bypass surgery. Remember, too, that pain in patients who have esophageal spasm or gallstones can occasionally mimic cardiac pain, but these patients rarely have the other signs and symptoms associated with cardiac disease. Jerry underscores these points in the 60-Second EMT Program."

> The 60-Second EMT should determine from the outset whether or not there is any history of cardiac disease.

Hawkins was getting to the center of things. "What do you mean by associated signs and symptoms?" I asked.

"These are very important," Hawkins stressed. "When Jerry encounters a patient with chest pain, he always asks about nausea, vomiting, sweating, syncope, palpitations, belching, involuntary

Symptoms that Point to Chest Pain of Cardiac Origin

nausea	belching
vomiting	involuntary defecation
sweating	shortness of breath
syncope	dyspnea on exertion
palpitations	nocturnal dyspnea

defecation, and shortness of breath. It's critical to know if nitro-glycerin relieved the pain and, if so, how many tablets were re-quired. The 60-Second EMT should also ask about dyspnea on exertion and nocturnal dyspnea. These symptoms strongly suggest that chest pain is of cardiac origin."

"Anything else?" I asked.

"Yes. Skin pallor, cyanosis, cool extremities, and tachypnea in-dicate severe cardiac failure," he added.

Donnelly made certain that the 60-Second EMT could paint a complete and detailed profile of myocardial infarction. I asked Hawkins what clues in the primary and secondary surveys helped the 60-Second EMT assess chest pain. Again, he was ready with answers.

"The patient's vital signs can give the 60-Second EMT an ex-traordinary amount of information," Hawkins informed me. "And what's so nice is that this information is available to the EMT very early in the encounter. Interpreting vital signs gives the 60-Second EMT a chance to shine."

"So how does the 60-Second EMT interpret the findings of the primary survey in patients with chest pain?" I asked.

"Well," began Hawkins as he continued his warm-up. "Within the first minute you know whether the pulse is regular or not. You know how fast or slow it is. A resting tachycardia is abnormal and might indicate mild heart failure or the stress from cardiac chest pain. A resting bradycardia is also abnormal and is sometimes seen with inferior wall infarction. An irregular pulse suggests some kind of cardiac abnormality. The most common cause is atrial fi-brillation. The blood pressure also can be revealing. A very low systolic pressure can indicate cardiogenic shock. Slightly elevated systolic and diastolic pressures are typical during the pain phase of myocardial infarction. Many EMTs and paramedics don't real-ize that mild hypertension is the rule in pulmonary edema. The respiratory rate can usually give you some idea of how much distress the patient is in. If dyspnea occurs in the setting of chest pain, congestive heart failure is likely; if there is severe respiratory distress and pinkish sputum, the patient probably has pulmonary edema."

"I guess you use the temperature to indicate infection," I offered.

"As a matter of fact, the absence or presence of fever can be very helpful," agreed Hawkins. "If the patient's temperature is above 102.5° F, then it's very likely that an infection is the cause of the patient's chest pain—in fact, all the P's in the CRAMPS mnemonic can cause fever. Remember, low-grade fever can also be seen with myocardial infarction, so it's not a perfect guide."

> If the patient's temperature is above 102.5° F, then it's very likely that an infection is the cause of the patient's chest pain.

It was extraordinary the way Donnelly had grouped chest pain into categories. I could see how the pain associated with myocardial infarction was very distinct from that associated with the other conditions. And I began to appreciate how data collected as part of the primary survey could help the EMT discriminate among the various causes of chest pain. There were still several issues I needed to resolve. I had seen many younger patients with chest pain and wondered whether the 60-Second EMT Exam had anything to offer this age group.

"What about chest pain in the young adult?" I queried. "You know the ones with chest wall pain?"

"Watch out. Young patients, especially those with a heavy smoking history or a family history of heart disease occurring at a young age, can have myocardial infarction."

"You're right," I admitted. "We've seen many heart attacks in men in the late 20s and early 30s–age group."

"But I think you're asking about the 'C' in CRAMPS—costochondritis and chest wall pain. These conditions are tricky and tough to assess," the runner said. "This group tends to be physically active; their chest pain can be caused by costochondritis or intercostal muscle strain. It's important to ask if there's been strenuous physical activity in the recent past. Usually, you can produce the pain by direct palpation over the chest wall."

"And what about anxiety and chest pain?"

"It's common, especially in young women," noted Hawkins. "These patients generally appear to be under stress and, frequently, they have other anxiety-related complaints such as dizziness, numbness and tingling of the extremities, lightheadedness, and hyperventilation."

"And I suppose they don't have the associated symptoms—nausea, diaphoreses, and such?"

"That's right. As a rule, they don't," Hawkins said. "Jerry likes to stress one thing though. These are diagnoses of exclusion. In other words, you can't be certain the patient in the field isn't having an MI, so you've always got to take *cardiac* precautions."

Hawkins had finished his warm-up and leaned over to tighten the shoelaces on his running shoes.

"Thanks for your time, Bill," I said.

"I'm glad I could help out," he answered. "And I hope you've gotten to know the 60-Second EMT a little better."

"I have," I said. "The 60-Second Chest Exam is a real feather in Donnelly's cap. That's for sure."

Just two days later, I was fortunate to again meet Bill Hawkins as he was warming up for his run.

"Bill, I just had to ask you if Jerry had integrated his 60-Second Chest Pain Assessment into the rapid assessment and intervention plans being adopted for acute MI."

Before I finished my sentence, Bill broke out in an ear-to-ear grin that even made me smile. He said, "I was waiting for you to ask me that. Just last week we responded to a fifty-five-year-old male who was having "the big one." He complained of retrosternal chest pain, which he described as a 'band squeezing my chest.' He said this pain had been present for 30 minutes and it radiated into his left arm, neck, and jaw. He was obviously pale, diaphoretic, and apprehensive."

"So, what did you and Jerry do?"

"We began by making sure the patient was sitting up to reduce the work required to breathe. This also helps if you suspect CHF. We immediately started nasal oxygen but were ready with a non–rebreather mask just in case. His vital signs were BP 154/96, pulse 68 and regular, respirations 24 and slightly labored, and SaO_2 of 93%. While I started a 16-gauge IV in a large forearm vein, Jerry auscultated his lungs, which were clear bilaterally.

> You can't be certain the patient in the field isn't having an MI, so always take *cardiac* precautions.

"As I hooked up the ECG, which showed sinus rhythm without ectopy, Jerry administered the first NTG tablet. We quickly moved the patient to the medic unit. In the medic unit, Jerry had me retake the BP as he administered another NTG and asked the patient if he had taken any medications that day or was allergic to aspirin. The patient denied either, so Jerry had him chew four baby aspirin tablets. Jerry told me that early ASA administration has been shown to greatly reduce post MI mortality. We continued to monitor and begin patient transport.

"I then saw Jerry pull out a checklist called the '60-Second EMT Thrombolytic Screening Sheet.' Jerry told me that if we could get certain information quickly, the hospital could make arrangements to immediately administer 'clot-busting' agents or arrange for emergency cardiac catheterization. While he asked our patient questions about stroke history, GI bleeds, recent head trauma, and recent surgeries, I hooked the patient up to the new 12-lead ECG machine.

"The 12-lead showed marked ST segment elevations in the anterior leads. The patient denied any history but still complained of pain. His vitals and ECG remained stable. As I administered the third NTG, Jerry contacted the hospital and advised them that we had a 10- to 15-minute ETA with a patient that was having an anterior MI who met the thrombolytic criteria. We had an ECG and checklist ready for the doc to review immediately upon arrival.

"We received authorization for IV nitroglycerin and morphine as needed and were told to secure a second large-bore IV as long as transport was not delayed. The ED physician was waiting when we arrived, and the nursing staff had already prepared the t-PA infusion. After reviewing the prehospital ECG and checklist, the physician ordered the t-PA started.

When EMTs collect appropriate information, physicians can quickly initiate advanced therapy.

"After we cleaned up, the ED physician stopped us and thanked us for obtaining this important information. He said that when EMTs collect appropriate information, physicians can quickly initiate advanced therapy. 'You guys probably saved his life.'

"So you see," Bill said, "the 60-Second EMT program is dynamic enough to encompass advances in prehospital care."

He took a deep breath and sprinted onto the track. He was as graceful as a gazelle as he rounded the first curve. As I watched him in the crisp autumn air I thought, "This is one guy who will never have chest pain."

Initial Therapy and Stabilization in Acute Myocardial Infarction

The diagnosis and treatment of acute myocardial infarction have become more sophisticated and interventional. Rapid assessment, identification, and intervention are essential to reducing mortality and morbidity in cardiac disease.

Where prehospital care fits is still being debated and studied. How much assessment should be done? What interventions are safe, cost effective, and clinically significant if performed in the field?

The following section presents several assessments and interventions that are appropriate for the patient with acute myocardial infarction. The appropriateness of each of them for the prehospital setting is system-dependant. EMS systems with identified needs, sound educational programs, and intense medical oversight may be the best qualified to provide such assessments and interventions.

General Approach: A team approach, based on communication between EMT and base station, is best suited for rapid assessment and therapeutic interventions that optimize outcomes in acute myocardial infarction. Any delay in providing therapy can cause unnecessary mortality and morbidity. Patients with suspected AMI should receive the following initial treatment and diagnostic monitoring:

STEP 1 PLACE PATIENT IN THE SITTING POSITION

Patients often wish to sit up; this increases tidal volume, decreases the work of breathing, and may improve symptoms of congestive heart failure and/or pulmonary edema.

STEP 2 OXYGENATION

All patients should be placed on supplemental oxygen. Monitor O_2 saturation by pulse oximetry, continuously if available, and maintain at $\geq 95\%$. The stable patient is placed on nasal-prong oxygen at flow rates of 2–4 L/min. Unstable patients are placed on 5–6 L/min by mask or 12–15 L/min. using a non–rebreather mask as needed to maintain O_2 sat at $\geq 95\%$. Continuous positive airway pressure (CPAP) applied with a tight-fitting mask also may improve oxygenation. If these efforts fail to maintain O_2 sat at $\geq 95\%$, arterial blood gases should be drawn and, if PO_2 is less than 60 mm Hg or acidosis is present, the patient should be endotracheally intubated and mechanically ventilated.

STEP 3 IV ACCESS

Two large-bore (16–18 gauge) lines should be secured. Antecubital sites are preferred if there are no large forearm veins.

STEP 4 CARDIAC AND BLOOD PRESSURE MONITORING

CARDIAC MONITOR: All patients should have a cardiac monitor applied.

BLOOD PRESSURE: Automatic blood pressure monitoring is available with some cardiac monitors and provides this critical information at frequent intervals. Initial values should be confirmed manually by mercury sphygmomanometer. BP should be measured in both arms if pain radiates to the back or legs or is associated with asymmetrically weak or absent upper-extremity pulses.

STEP 5 INITIAL MANAGEMENT OF CHEST PAIN

PAIN RELIEF: Mortality reduction in AMI has not been demonstrated for either sublingual nitroglycerin or morphine sulphate intravenously. Despite this, these agents are the initial-treatment standard of practice because of the clinical benefits of preload reduction and pain relief.

Sublingual Nitroglycerin: Administer 0.3- or 0.4-mg tablet (Nitrostat) or 0.4-mg spray (Nitrolingual) every 5 minutes if the BP remains above 110 mm Hg. In these doses nitroglycerin causes preload reduction by venodialation. If symptoms are not relieved with three doses, particularly if there is no change with the first two, IV nitroglycerin should be prepared and IV morphine sulphate should be given. 2% to 3% of patients given sublingual nitroglyerin will experience hypotension due to hypovolemia and/or right ventricular infarction. After intravenous normal saline correction of the hypotension, ECG with leads V_3R and V_4R should be obtained to rule out right ventricular infarction (16). Rarely, symptomatic sinus bradycardia may occur and may be treated with atropine (see Bradycardia). For persistent chest pain, hypertension, or pulmonary rales: IV nitroglycerin: if BP is > 110 systolic, start at 10–20 µg/min; advance to 50–180 µg/min increments of 5–10 µg/min every 5 minutes.

STEP 6 ADDITIONAL THERAPY FOR CHEST PAIN

IV MORPHINE: Administer 2–4 mg every 5 to 10 minutes as needed for pain if the BP remains above 110 mm Hg systolic. Complications of morphine include hypotension, treated with normal saline infusion; nausea and vomiting, treated with discontinuation of the drug; itching at the site, treated with discontinuation and, in the uncommon event of generalized itching, diphenhydramine (Benadryl), 25–50 mg intravenously. Symptomatic sinus bradycardia is treated with atropine if persistent. Respiratory depression rarely occurs but the effects of morphine can be reversed by naloxone (Narcan) in small doses of 0.1–0.2 mg IV to avoid sudden analgesic withdrawal. Pulse oximetry and blood pressure should be monitored carefully during such episodes.

Myocardial Salvage and Mortality Reduction in Acute Myocardial Infarction

After initial stabilization has been performed, the following four interventional strategies should be considered in all patients who have chest pain and/or a clinical presentation strongly suspicious of acute myocardial infarction (AMI).

INTERVENTION PHASE 1: ASPIRIN

Because of the dramatic benefits and minimal risk associated with aspirin therapy, virtually all patients with suspected MI who have no contraindications to the use of salicylates should receive this agent.

Administer:

ASPIRIN (ASA)

325 mg: 4 baby aspirin tablets or one adult aspirin tablet, chew and swallow; if vomiting is present, 325 mg suppository per rectum.

- ENTRY CRITERIA REQUIRED FOR ASA ADMINISTRATION:
  Clinical Suspicion of Acute Myocardial Infarction.
    ECG confirmation of AMI not required.
    No age limit.
- TIME FRAME:
  Administer ASA up to 24 hours or more after onset of symptoms.
- EXCLUSIONARY CRITERIA:
  Allergy to ASA.

INTERVENTION PHASE 2: THROMBOLYTIC AGENTS

Thrombolysis plays a pivotal role in myocardial salvage and mortality reduction in acute myocardial infarction. To maximize cost-effectiveness and benefit/risk ratio, patients should meet the entry and exclusionary criteria outlined below. The choice of thrombolytic agents in this guideline has included consideration of both cost and evidentiary studies demonstrating relative advantages of one agent versus another in specific patient subgroups.

Administer:

STREPTOKINASE 1.5 million U IV over one hour:

Preferred Thrombolytic Agent

In patients >75 years of age with inferior or lateral MI, with chest pain symptoms for more than 4 hours,

or, as an alternative:

ACCELERATED t-PA WITH IV HEPARIN

For patients <75, anterior AMI, and symptoms under 4 hours (GUSTO):

t-PA: a) 15 mg bolus.
   b) 0.75 mg/kg up to 50 mg over 30 minutes.
   c) 0.5 mg/kg up to 35 mg over 60 minutes.

Heparin: 5000 U IV bolus and 1000 U/hour (1200 U if > 80 kg);
   keep PTT in the 60–85–second range.

or Standard t-PA: 100 mg over 3 hours IV
   (GISSI-2/International Study Group).

or Standard APSAC: 30 U over 3 minutes IV (ISIS-3).

- ENTRY CRITERIA FOR THROMBOLYSIS:
  1) No age limit.
  2) Killip class I and II only.

- TIME FRAME:
  Up to 12 hours from onset of symptoms; or up to 24 hours of symptoms in patients with stuttering pattern of symptoms.

- ECG CRITERIA:
  Obtain leads V_{3R} and V_{4R} when inferior or lateral changes are present:
  a) ST-Elevation: >1 mm in two contiguous leads (GISSI-2).
  b) Any of the following with strong clinical history: LBBB, pathologic Q waves >2 mm, T-wave inversion, II° or III°AV block, any arrhythmia (ISIS-2).

- LIMITATION CRITERIA:
  Prior exposure to APSAC or streptokinase or recent streptococcal infection; Only t-PA is appropriate.

- EXCLUSIONARY CRITERIA:
  Note: If aortic dissection is suspected, perform immediate CT scan of thorax with contrast or transesophageal echocardiography.
  For patients who are excluded from thrombolysis because of one or more of the exclusionary criteria listed below: CONSIDER IMMEDIATE CORONARY ANGIOPLASTY (PTCA).
  1. History of stroke or TIA in past 6 months.
  2. Recent head trauma or known intracranial mass.
  3. Surgery, PTCA, or severe trauma in last 2 weeks.
  4. Recent GI bleed or ulcer.
  5. BP >110 diastolic, >200 systolic, persistent despite IV NTG.
  6. Noncompressible venous or arterial puncture.
  7. History of bleeding disorder or anticoagulation.
  8. Cardiopulmonary resuscitation > 10 minutes (relative contraindication).
  9. Pulmonary edema and/or cardiogenic shock (Killip class III or IV).
  10. Pericarditis.
  11. Pregnancy.

INTERVENTION PHASE 3: BETA-BLOCKADE

Beta-blockade has been shown to improve mortality following MI, with patients greater than 65 years of age deriving the most benefit (ISIS-1). It is especially useful in patients with MI who have recurrent symptoms of ischemia, hypertension, or sinus tachycardia.

Administer:

ATENOLOL

5 mg IV q 10 min to a total of 10 mg followed in 15 minutes by 50 mg po as tolerated,

or

METOPROLOL

5 mg IV q 5–10 min to a total of 15 mg followed in 15 minutes by 100 mg po as tolerated.

- ENTRY CRITERIA
    1. Clinical stability after thrombolytic agent (BP >110, no wheezes).
    2. Killip class I only: no evidence of congestive heart failure.
- EXCLUSIONARY CRITERIA
    1. Asthma (as an adult) or COPD.
    2. AV block.
    3. Hypotension (BP < 100).
    4. Congestive heart failure.

INTERVENTION PHASE 4: ACE INHIBITORS

Angiotensin Converting Enzyme (ACE) Inhibitors have been shown (ISIS-4) to produce minimal to modest improvements in mortality following MI.

Administer:

LISINOPRIL

BP > 120: 5 mg orally q 24 hours.

BP ≤ 120: 2.5 mg orally q 24 hours (GISSI-3).

CAPTOPRIL

(ISIS-4)

- ENTRY CRITERION
    1. Killip class I and II.
- EXCLUSIONARY CRITERIA
    1. Allergy to ACEIs.
    2. Killip class III and IV.
    3. History of renal failure, bilateral renal artery stenosis.

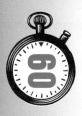
CHEST PAIN

CRAMPS	P PROVOCATIVE	PALLIATIVE	Q QUALITY
Costochondritis	Respirations Movement Palpation Cough	Shallow breathing Splinting	Sharp
Rebound pain (same as for Myocardial infarction)			
Aneurysm	None	None	Deep tearing
Anxiety	Stress Stimulants	Relaxation	Sharp, occasion
Myocardial infarction	None	None	Crushing Heavy Dull pressing Band-like
Pneumonia	Respirations Cough	Shallow breathing	Sharp or dull a
Pericarditis	Supine posture Respirations Cough	Upright posture Shallow breathing	Sharp
Pneumothorax	Respirations Cough	None	Sharp
Pleurisy	Respirations Cough	Shallow breathing	Sharp
Spasm (Esophageal)	Supine (delayed) posture	Antacids	Dull pressing Collicky

	R		S	T
ION	**RADIATION**	**SEVERITY**		**TIME**
ior & lateral	Locally	(+)−+++		After exercise Subacute onset
ernal	Back	(++++)		Sudden onset May subside spontaneously
s in chest	Usually none	(+)−(++)		Subacute onset
ernal (can vary)	Jaw Either arm	(+)−++++		After exercise Heavy meals Stress with SOB With nausea and sweating
lly	None	(+)−(++)		With fever, cough Slow onset
ernally	Usually none, occasional tip of shoulder	(+)−(+++)		Subacute onset
lly	None	+−+++		Sudden onset, after exercise, may subside with SOB
lly	None	+−+++		Subacute onset with flu symptoms
ernally, tric	Jaw, either arm	(+)−(++)		Subacute onset after meals, at night with acid taste

THROMBOLYTIC THERAPY CHECKLIST

INCLUSIONS: (MUST ANSWER "YES" TO ALL)

1. Is the patient between 18 and 75 years old?   Y   N
2. Has the patient had chest pain for <6 hours?   Y   N
3. Is the pain not relieved by sublingual NTG?   Y   N
4. Does the 12-lead ECG show ST elevation of 1 mm or greater in 2 contiguous leads?   Y   N

EXCLUSIONS: (MUST ANSWER "NO" TO ALL)

1. Does the patient have history of stroke/TIA within 6 months?   Y   N
2. Does the patient have history of surgery, PCTA, or severe trauma within 2 weeks?   Y   N
3. Has the patient had recent GI bleeding or ulcer?   Y   N
4. Has there been recent head trauma or intercranial mass?   Y   N
5. Is there a history of bleeding disorder?   Y   N
6. Does the patient have pulmonary edema, pericarditis, or pleural effusion?   Y   N
7. Is the patient pregnant?   Y   N

Notes: Items 1 and 2 of the inclusion criteria are relative. Consider also older patients who lead active lifestyles, especially if the onset of pain is recent. The 6-hour time window is also relative. If the patient seeks care within 12 hours, the physician may still wish to proceed with thrombolytic treatment.

If the patient is excluded from thrombolysis because of one or more of the above, advise the hospital to stand by for urgent PCTA.

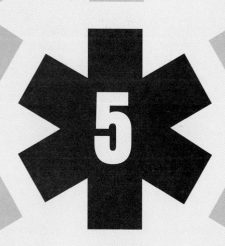

5

The 60-Second Special Lecture: Code Blue

n addition to his renown as an EMT, Jerry Donnelly has quite a reputation as an educator. One of our paramedics, Katelyn Cohen, attended a lecture that Donnelly gave on the new ACLS guidelines. She started describing some of the things she had learned.

"Jerry told us some interesting things about giving meds. He said that if meds are administered through a peripheral line, we should follow up with a 20-ml fluid bolus and elevate the extremity."

Well, it made sense to me. Just as I was getting really interested in hearing more, Katelyn said that she had to be going. On her way to the door she handed me a copy of her lecture notes.

Code Blue

Introduction

In the fall of 1992 the American Heart Association published new recommendations for advanced cardiac life support (ACLS). The revised standards reflect not only review of previous standards but recent research in basic science and clinical trials. Also included are a grading of risk versus benefit for the ACLS interventions and encouragement for medical personnel in the use of clinical skills and judgment in resuscitation.

Emphasis to the general public and prehospital care personnel is on the chain of survival. Links in this chain are early access of EMS, early CPR, early defibrillation, and early ACLS.

Adult Emergency Cardiac Care

New to the ACLS teaching and care algorithms is the universal algorithm for adult emergency cardiac care (see algorithm on next page). This is a combination of BLS and an entry into the specific treatment algorithms.

The Chain of Survival

| early access to EMS | early CPR | early defibrillation | early ACLS |

UNIVERSAL ALGORITHM FOR ADULT EMERGENCY CARDIAC CARE

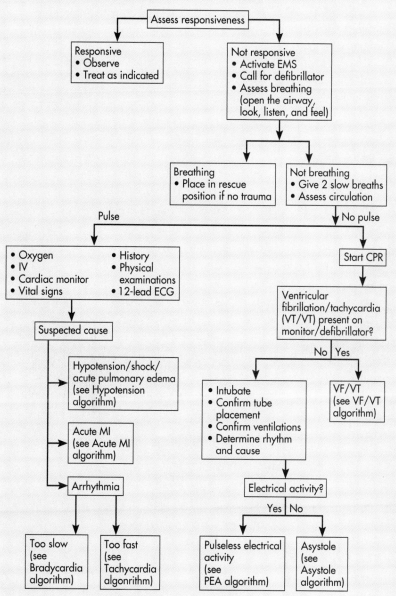

ALGORITHM FOR PULSELESS ELECTRICAL ACTIVITY (PEA)

PEA includes
- Electromechanical dissociation (EMD)
- Pseudo-EMD
- Idioventricular rhythms
- Ventricular escape rhythms
- Bradyasystolic rhythms
- Postdefibrillation idioventricular rhythms

- Continue CPR
- Intubate at once

- Obtain IV access
- Assess blood flow using Doppler ultrasound

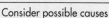

Consider possible causes
(Parentheses = possible therapies and treatments)
- Hypovolemia (volume infusion)
- Hypoxia (ventilation)
- Cardiac tamponade (pericardiocentesis)
- Tension pneumothorax (needle decompression)
- Hypothermia
- Massive pulmonary embolism (surgery, thrombolytics)
- Drug overdoses such as tricyclics, digitalis, β-blockers, calcium channel blockers
- Hyperkalemia
- Acidosis
- Massive acute myocardial infarction

- Epinephrine 1 mg IV push, repeat every 3-5 min

- If absolute bradycardia (<60 beats/min) or relative bradycardia, give atropine 1 mg IV
- Repeat every 3-5 min up to a total of 0.04 mg/kg

---

cardiac tamponade, tension pneumothorax, and severe acidosis. New considerations are cardiodepressant drug overdose, hyperkalemia, and massive MI. If found early, hyperkalemia will respond to sodium bicarbonate and calcium.

Epinephrine remains the first-line drug. The dose remains 1 mg

Classification of Therapeutic Interventions in CPR and ECC

Class I—Usually indicated, always acceptable, and considered useful and effective.
Class IIa—Acceptable, *probably* beneficial.
Class IIb—Acceptable, *possibly* beneficial.
Class III—Inappropriate, may be harmful.

From: JAMA 1992 p. 2174.

IV. High-dose regimens of epinephrine are included in the protocol as Class IIb recommendations. Atropine has been added to the PEA protocol for true or relative bradycardic nonperfusing rhythms.

Asystole Treatment

The asystole algorithm (see below) has not significantly changed. The protocol strongly encourages considering a differential diagnosis for asystole, including checking lead placement and equipment. Hypoxia, potassium disorders, severe acidosis, and hypothermia should be considered also.

The use of transcutaneous pacing (TCP) should be considered and, if chosen, should be started at the earliest possible time. The hope is that if cardiac arrest is caused by deteriorating bradycardia, early use of TCP may provide capture. In the past it was suggested that defibrillation of asystole was acceptable under the possibility of fine VF. This is no longer recommended because defibrillation may increase parasympathetic tone, which,

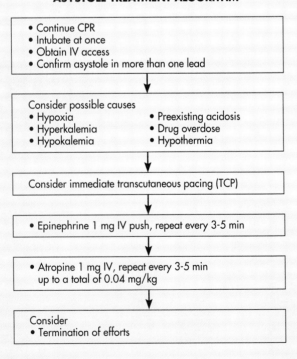

ASYSTOLE TREATMENT ALGORITHM

- Continue CPR
- Intubate at once
- Obtain IV access
- Confirm asystole in more than one lead

↓

Consider possible causes
- Hypoxia
- Hyperkalemia
- Hypokalemia
- Preexisting acidosis
- Drug overdose
- Hypothermia

↓

Consider immediate transcutaneous pacing (TCP)

↓

- Epinephrine 1 mg IV push, repeat every 3-5 min

↓

- Atropine 1 mg IV, repeat every 3-5 min up to a total of 0.04 mg/kg

↓

Consider
- Termination of efforts

in true asystole, renders the heart less responsive to atropine and, possibly, epinephrine. Drug therapy remains epinephrine in 1-mg increments. High-dose epinephrine is acceptable but probably not helpful. Atropine is given in 1-mg increments repeated every 3 to 5 minutes, to a total dose of 0.04 mg/kg, which is 3 mg in an average-sized adult (70-75 kg).

The protocols also address prearrest conditions: bradycardia, tachycardias, acute MI, and hypotension with congestive heart failure and pulmonary edema. The starting point for treatment in all of these conditions is an assessment of stability and patient tolerance.

Bradycardia

For bradycardic rhythms, instability consists of chest pain, shortness of breath, decreased level of consciousness or measured parameters of low blood pressure, CHF, or ventricular ectopy. For patients who are stable, the treatment is the same as before—observation only. For higher degree (second type II, or third degree) observation and placement of transcutaneous pacer (if available) are recommended.

The treatment for symptomatic bradycardia has changed (see algorithm on next page). For all bradycardias requiring treatment, TCP is a Class I intervention. For low-degree heart block, atropine is recommended as first-line therapy in a dosage range of 0.5- to 1.0-mg increments, to a total dose of 0.04 mg/kg. For high-degree heart block with wide complex ventricular escape rhythms, atropine is discouraged and pacing is the recommended first intervention, if available. If atropine is ineffective, catecholamine infusion is the next therapy. Isoproterenol is no longer recommended. Dopamine infusion at a rate of 5-20 ucg/kg/min is recommended titrated to patient response. If the patient is severely bradycardic and hypotensive, epinephrine infusion is recommended. The dose is 2-10 ucg/min. This treatment can be thought of as restoring the patient's PEA level to the point at which pharmacologic intervention can be epinephrine. One caveat added to the algorithm is that if the patient has had cardiac transplantation, he or she will not respond to atropine regardless of the rhythm.

Tachycardia

For tachycardic rhythms, treatment begins with assessment of stability. For stable patients, initial therapy consists of

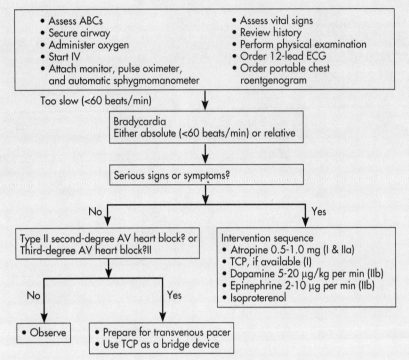

BRADYCARDIA ALGORITHM

- Assess ABCs
- Secure airway
- Administer oxygen
- Start IV
- Attach monitor, pulse oximeter, and automatic sphygmomanometer

- Assess vital signs
- Review history
- Perform physical examination
- Order 12-lead ECG
- Order portable chest roentgenogram

Too slow (<60 beats/min)

Bradycardia
Either absolute (<60 beats/min) or relative

Serious signs or symptoms?

No

Type II second-degree AV heart block? or Third-degree AV heart block?II

No   Yes

- Observe

- Prepare for transvenous pacer
- Use TCP as a bridge device

Yes

Intervention sequence
- Atropine 0.5-1.0 mg (I & IIa)
- TCP, if available (I)
- Dopamine 5-20 µg/kg per min (IIb)
- Epinephrine 2-10 µg per min (IIb)
- Isoproterenol

medication administration. Unstable patients receive synchronized cardioversion.* For borderline patients, a trial of medication can be used. (If the patient is conscious, consider sedation). The sequence for cardioversion has been expanded to four countershocks at 100, 200, 300, and 360 joules. If there is brief conversion at a lower energy, it should be used on the subsequent shock. Monitor diagnosis should be made for atrial fibrillation and atrial flutter, PSVT, wide complex tachycardia (WCT), and VT.

Atrial Fibrillation

Treatment of atrial fibrillation and atrial flutter consists of medications that control ventricular response: calcium channel

---

* Severely unstable patients (unconscious, with pulmonary edema or profound hypotension) receive immediate, unsynchronized cardioversion.

blockers, beta-blockers, digoxin, procainamide, or quinidine. No patients should receive intravenous calcium channel blockade and beta-blockade together. For treatment of tolerated PSVT, adenosine has replaced verapamil. The dose is 6 mg IV push as rapidly as possible followed by saline flush. Conversion should occur in 15-30 seconds. If unsuccessful, repeat dosing with 12 mg.

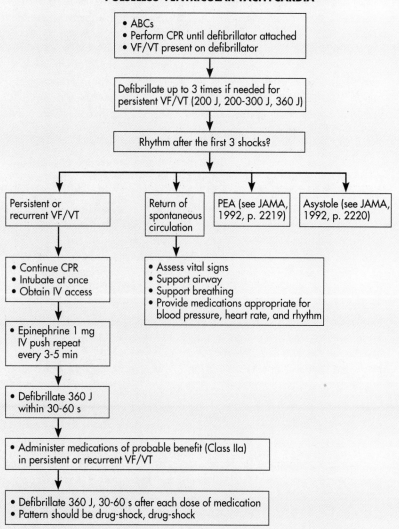

ALGORITHM FOR VENTRICULAR FIBRILLATION AND PULSELESS VENTRICULAR TACHYCARDIA

- ABCs
- Perform CPR until defibrillator attached
- VF/VT present on defibrillator

Defibrillate up to 3 times if needed for persistent VF/VT (200 J, 200-300 J, 360 J)

Rhythm after the first 3 shocks?

| Persistent or recurrent VF/VT | Return of spontaneous circulation | PEA (see JAMA, 1992, p. 2219) | Asystole (see JAMA, 1992, p. 2220) |

Persistent or recurrent VF/VT:
- Continue CPR
- Intubate at once
- Obtain IV access

- Epinephrine 1 mg IV push repeat every 3-5 min

- Defibrillate 360 J within 30-60 s

- Administer medications of probable benefit (Class IIa) in persistent or recurrent VF/VT

- Defibrillate 360 J, 30-60 s after each dose of medication
- Pattern should be drug-shock, drug-shock

Return of spontaneous circulation:
- Assess vital signs
- Support airway
- Support breathing
- Provide medications appropriate for blood pressure, heart rate, and rhythm

Verapamil is reserved only for narrow complex normotensive patients.

Precise diagnosis of the rhythms of patients with WCT can be a challenge. The new recommendations take this into account. If the patient is unstable, treatment consists of cardioversion. Initial drug therapy is with lidocaine 1-1.5 mg/kg with repeat if needed of 0.5-0.75 mg/kg, to a total dose of 3 mg/kg. Adenosine may be tried next. This should be successful if the rhythm is supraventricular. Verapamil is not to be used for WCT if there is any possibility of the rhythms being ventricular in origin. Treatment of known ventricular tachycardia should be cardioversion if the patient is unstable, and medication if he or she is stable (see algorithm on previous page). Initial therapy is lidocaine at the same dosage as in WCT, followed by procainamide, followed by bretylium, followed by cardioversion if there is not conversion with drug therapy.

No patients should receive intravenous calcium channel blockade and beta-blockade together.

An additional algorithm in the new standards is hypotension/shock/acute pulmonary edema. After initial evaluation and assessment, the next step is to determine the nature of the problem. Stop and think before beginning therapy. The cardiovascular triad is used as a guiding "tool": Is this a rate problem, a pump problem, or a volume problem?

If the problem is rate, treatment should follow the bradycardia or tachycardia algorithm. Hemodynamic monitoring is useful for determining volume status and pump status; but history, examination, and clinical judgment can give an accurate impression. Volume problems can be absolute, as in blood loss or fluid loss, or can be relative because of vascular collapse. Initial treatment is fluid challenge; if there is a vascular tone problem, pressors can be added. Determining this may require invasive monitoring.

Pump Problems

Pump problems can be caused by infarction, valvular disease, or ineffective cardiac action from drugs, hypoxia, or poisoning. A fluid challenge is appropriate, 250-500 cc, if pulmonary edema is not present. For pump failure with severe hypotension, that is, a systolic BP of 70 or less, norepinephrine should be first-line therapy at 0.5-30 ucg/min titrated to response. Dopamine should

ACUTE MYOCARDIAL INFARCTION ALGORITHM

Community
- Community emphasis on "call first/call fast, call 911"
- National Heart Attack Alert Program

↓

EMS System
EMS system approach that should address
- Oxygen-IV-cardiac monitor-vital signs
- Nitroglycerin
- Pain relief with narcotics
- Notification of emergency department
- Rapid transport to emergency department
- Prehospital screening for thrombolytic therapy*
- 12-lead ECG, computer analysis, transmission to emergency department*
- Initiation of thrombolytic therapy*

↓

Emergency Department
"Door-to-drug" team protocol approach
- Rapid triage of patients with chest pain
- Clinical decision maker established (emergency physician, cardiologist, or other)

| Time interval in emergency department |

↓

Assessment immediate:	Treatments to consider if there is evidence of coronary thrombosis plus no reasons for exclusion (some but not all may be appropriate)
• Vital signs with automatic BP	• Oxygen at 4 L/min
• Oxygen saturation	• Nitroglycerin SL, paste or spray (if systolic blood pressure >90 mm Hg)
• Start IV	• Morphine IV
• 12-lead ECG (MD review)	• Aspirin PO
• Brief, targeted history and physical	• Thrombolytic agents
• Decide on eligibility for thrombolytic therapy	• Nitroglycerin IV (limit systolic BP drop to 10% if normotensive; 30% drop if hypertensive; never drop below 90 mm Hg systolic)
Soon:	• ß-Blockers IV
• Chest roentgenogram	• Heparin IV
• Blood studies (electrolytes, enzymes, coagulation studies)	• Percutaneous transluminal coronary angioplasty
• Consult as needed	• Routine lidocaine administration is not recommended for all
*Optional guidelines	patients with AMI

| 30-60 min to thrombolytic therapy |

be used for hypotension but only with systolic pressures above 70. First-line therapy for pulmonary edema has been added to the algorithm and remains as taught in the past in use of morphine, sublingual nitroglycerin, and Lasix. IV nitroglycerin is also recommended as an early intervention. These interventions are for the normotensive or hypertensive patient with pulmonary edema.

Uncomplicated MI

A final algorithm is for the treatment of uncomplicated MI (note algorithm on previous page). This protocol consists of the ABCs of ACLS: initiation of oxygen, monitoring, and IV access, as well as prehospital drug therapy with nitroglycerin and morphine as needed for pain relief and transport. For services with long transport times and ability to transmit EKGs, prehospital initiation of thrombolytic agents is a possibility. For routine MI without high-risk ectopy, lidocaine prophylaxis is no longer recommended. (See Chapter 4 for in-depth discussion of MI intervention).

Conclusion

The new protocols have been changed. These therapeutic changes are based on current research and should make treatment simpler and more effective. Emergency medical personnel are encouraged to use their own clinical judgment. They will be helped by the new grading for the effectiveness of various interventions, as they consider causes of instability and collapse and incorporate these in their treatment plans.

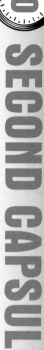

CODE BLUE

- The ABCs are still of prime importance.
- Immediate assessment should be made for Vfib/VTach: immediate defibrillation is indicated upon recognition. 200/200-300/360 sequence is still used; pulse checks are no longer needed between "stacked shocks."
- Epinephrine 1.0 mg over 3-5 minutes is first-drug of choice for all cardiac arrest patients. "High-dose" Epi is optional.
- EMD is renamed pulseless electrical activity (PEA). Direct efforts toward ABC and treating the cause. Atropine should be given in PEA with bradycardia.
- Atropine is questionable for infranodal AV blocks. Transcutaneous pacing (TCP) is the initial treatment of choice.
- Adenosine is Class I for stable adult supraventricular tachycardia.
- Epinephrine and atropine should be given close together for asystole. Shorter time intervals may be helpful.

PHYSICAL FINDINGS IN PEA

1. Venous pooling in arrest situation should cause neck vein distention. Flat neck veins indicate consideration of decreased volume.
2. Jugular venous distention plus tracheal deviation plus decreased breath sounds indicate consideration of tension pneumothorax.
3. Decreased breath sounds, especially on the left side, indicate examination of tube placement.
4. Breath sounds over the stomach indicate examination of tube placement.
5. Jugular venous distention and midline trachea and non-chest trauma indicate consideration of cardiac tamponade.
6. Jugular venous distention, recent surgery, or immobilization and blue skin color indicate consideration of pulmonary embolus.

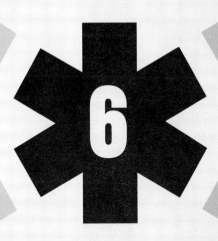

6

The 60-Second Abdominal Assessment

ynne Harkness was an emergency nurse, EMT-P, and the EMT training coordinator for the hospital at which Jerry Donnelly was based. Lynne and Jerry had developed a quality-assurance program for prehospital care providers based at their hospital. Twice a month Harkness led a citywide conference to discuss problem cases whose reports had filtered up to the head of the county's EMS system. After five years of caring for patients in a busy emergency department and three years out in the field, Harkness was uniquely qualified to shed light on the 60-Second EMT Program that she had adopted for the EMTs attending her teaching conference.

The night before our meeting, Lynne told me over the phone that she was looking forward to telling me about Donnelly's 60-second approach to the assessment and triage of abdominal pain. She said that almost everyone she knew—whether physicians, paramedics, or EMTs—felt some insecurity about the diagnosis, evaluation, and triage of patients with abdominal pain. From what I could gather, Donnelly and Harkness had put together a systematic approach for managing this group of patients. In fact, she was so happy with the results that she had created an audiocassette/slide program for the 60-Second Abdominal Exam. She told me that she would bring it to our meeting for a "private screening."

We met in the hospital auditorium, a newly built conference facility with a state-of-the-art audiovisual system. I walked into the auditorium and noticed Lynne's notebook on a seat near the back of the auditorium. I looked up at the AV booth and saw Lynne loading a carousel onto the projector. The room lights dimmed. As I sat down, the screen filled with a crisp blue-on-black slide that read, "The 60-Second Assessment of Abdominal Pain, by Lynne Harkness and Jerry Donnelly."

Without warning, Lynne bounced into the seat next to mine and, with a smile that lit the darkness, said, "It's not fine filmmaking, but I think you'll get what you're after." She pressed the button on her remote unit and advanced the carousel to the next slide, which read

ABDOMINAL PAIN SYNDROMES: RAPID ASSESSMENT & TRIAGE

"I love these remote control slide projectors," she said. "Maybe it's because they remind me of watching TV."

Her free-spirited disposition and upbeat mannerisms reminded me of watching TV, or, rather, someone on TV. Katie Couric of "NBC" crossed my mind.

"I appreciate your taking the time to give this slide talk," I said by way of introduction. "I'm sure you've heard that I've spoken with a lot of people about Donnelly's 60-Second EMT Program. You're the only one who's actually put one of the training modules into a show-and-tell format."

"Actually, this slide show is a prototype," explained Harkness. "Jerry and I plan to package all the modules in the 60-Second EMT Program into a comprehensive audiocassette/slide program. There's been a tremendous demand for it from instructors and co-ordinators all over the country." Lynne projected the next slide, which had bright red-on-black lettering. It read,

ABDOMINAL PAIN: PRESENTATIONS

"Jerry stresses the many different ways in which abdominal conditions, life-threatening or not, can be present. The 60-Second EMT has to have a complete grasp of the physical signs, symptoms, and historical features associated with abdominal pain, or serious assessment mistakes are inevitable."

The next slide appeared, with the following syndromes listed:

BACK PAIN, PERITONEAL SYMPTOMS, COLICKY PAIN SYNDROMES, VOMITING SYNDROMES, HEMORRHAGIC SYNDROMES, GYNECOLOGIC DISORDERS

"You see, any of these presentations is consistent with an abdominal catastrophe of some kind or another," explained Harkness, clicking the button on the remote unit.

The next slide appeared on the screen. Bright red letters spelled out,

BACK PAIN: WATCH OUT!

"I'm sure you know the significance of this slide," she said.

"I assume you're trying to call attention to the fact that several life-threatening abdominal disorders can have back pain as their most prominent symptom."

"That's right," Harkness confirmed. "Look at this next slide. It

Causes of Abdominal Pain in the Elderly	
Abdominal pain of unknown etiology	Duodenal ulcer
Constipation	Aortic abdominal aneurysm
Cholelithiasis	Appendicitis
Acute cholecystitis	Mesenteric ischemia
Intestinal obstruction	Obstructive uropathy
Acute pancreatitis	Volvulus
Gastroenteritis	

lists all the abdominal conditions that can produce back pain as the patient's presenting chief complaint."

I studied the list, which included abdominal aortic aneurysm, pancreatitis, cholecystitis, and perforated peptic ulcer.

"In an elderly patient without a history of trauma," Lynne continued, "EMTs should consider abdominal aortic aneurysm as a possible diagnosis. A history of high blood pressure combined with a presenting low pressure and a pulsating abdominal mass on physical exam is a tip-off. Diminished femoral pulses are also a key physical finding. I can't tell you how many times Jerry and I have suspected—and then made—the diagnosis of abdominal aneurysm in elderly patients who had suddenly developed excruciating back pain for no apparent reason."

> In an elderly patient without a history of trauma, consider abdominal aortic aneurysm.

"If the history and physical strongly suggest an aneurysm, I suppose you put in an IV line and transport Code 3?"

"That's right," she said. "Now look at the other conditions on the list. Gallstones, for example, can produce a variety of symptoms, including back pain. Usually, it is accompanied by nausea and vomiting, and, not uncommonly, back pain can be the presenting symptom. This isn't always the case, of course. Most of the time, the patient with gallstones, known as cholelithiasis, has right-upper-quadrant pain after eating a fatty meal, along with severe nausea and vomiting. If fever is present with these symptoms, you have to worry about cholecystitis, which is inflammation of the gallbladder sac. The discomfort is called 'colicky' pain. That's coming up in a few slides."

> Gallstones can produce a variety of symptoms, including back pain.

"You know, Lynne," I said. "I think this approach is very use-

Common Anatomic Pain Sites for Specific Causes of Acute Abdominal Pain

RIGHT UPPER QUADRANT AND FLANK

Cholecystitis   Intestinal obstruction
Pyelonephritis   Retrocecal appendicitis
Penetrating ulcer   Pancreatitis
Choledocholithiasis   Gastric ulcer

EPIGASTRIUM

Pancreatitis   Gastritis
Duodenal ulcer   Early appendicitis
Penetrating ulcer   Mesenteric ischemia
Colon carcinoma   Abdominal aortic aneurysm

LEFT UPPER QUADRANT AND FLANK

Splenic enlargement   Diverticulitis
Pyelonephritis   Bowel obstruction
Splenic rupture

RIGHT LOWER QUADRANT

Appendicitis   Bowel obstruction
Hernia   Pyelonephritis
Cholecystitis   Diverticulitis
Psoas abscess   Leaking aneurysm
Ectopic pregnancy

LEFT LOWER QUADRANT

Diverticulitis   Bowel obstruction
Hernia   Leaking aneurysm
Pyelonephritis   Abdominal wall hematoma
Ectopic pregnancy

HYPOGASTRIUM

Diveriticulitis   Cystitis
Bladder obstruction   Appendicitis
Prostatism   Hernia
Bowel obstruction   Colon carcinoma

ful. Too often paramedics write off back pain as a manifestation of arthritis or lumbosacral muscle strain. Obviously, that can be very dangerous. The 60-Second Abdominal Assessment stresses the importance of considering abdominal causes of back pain. I like that.''

''There are two more important abdominal conditions that can produce back pain as the predominant feature,'' Lynne continued as she pressed the button on her remote unit. ''The first is pancreatitis, and the second is a perforated peptic ulcer. The uncanny thing about a perforated ulcer is that the patient can usually tell you exactly—sometimes, even to the minute—when the pain began. That's because perforation is so painful and causes generalized peritoneal inflammation. When the EMT suspects perforation, he or she should try to elicit a history of ulcer disease, aspirin, ibuprofen or nonsteroid anti-inflammatory drug (NSAID) use, or recent flare-up of ulcer symptoms."

"Are these the kinds of patients that have a stiff, board-like abdomen?" I inquired.

"Very often they do, but not always," Lynne answered, advancing the slide to

PANCREATITIS

"Finally, there's pancreatitis," she explained. "As a rule, abdominal pain with radiation to the back is the chief complaint, but, on occasion, back pain is the main symptom. Alcoholics, elderly patients with gallstones, and those with ulcer disease are at risk for pancreatitis. People with this condition frequently sit up and double over on the stretcher. It seems to ease the pain."

The next slide filled the screen. It said,

COLICKY PAIN VS. PERITONEAL PAIN: KNOW THE DIFFERENCE!

"This is a key part of the 60-Second Abdominal Exam," Lynne explained, "because there are different pain syndromes associated with different abdominal structures. Jerry makes sure that EMTs in his 60-second program know what the assessment implications are for each type of pain syndrome."

"What exactly do you mean by pain syndrome?" I asked.

"Look here," she said, advancing the slide.

COLICKY PAIN: AN INTENSE SPASMODIC PAIN CAUSED BY SMOOTH MUSCLE CONTRACTIONS IN A HOLLOW VISCOUS ORGAN AGAINST A MECHANICAL OBSTRUCTION.

"Colicky pain is just what this slide says it is," said Lynne. "It's an intense spasm—really intense. It's the kind of pain that makes the patient writhe all over the stretcher. The pain has a roller-coaster quality. At the outset it comes in waves, but as the condition progresses the pain may become constant. It can be very intense and then subside, only to return with even more force. Not uncommonly, the pain is severe enough to produce vomiting."

The next slide came into focus:

CAUSES OF COLICKY PAIN: [1] SMALL OR LARGE BOWEL
OBSTRUCTION: ADHESIONS, SIGMOID VOLVULUS, OR NEOPLASM;
[2] BILE DUCT OBSTRUCTION: GALLSTONES, PANCREATITIS, ULCER
DISEASE; [3] OBSTRUCTION OF THE URETERS: KIDNEY DISEASE.

"That clears things up a bit," I said, realizing that this slide attempted to highlight abdominal structures that could cause colicky pain.

"I think it's a nice approach too, not only for EMTs and paramedics but for the nurses in my department." Lynne offered. "When you see a patient writhing on the stretcher and he or she tells you the pain is coming in waves or spasms, you know you have to consider one of these colicky pain syndromes. It's also important to remember that, as a rule, palpation of the abdomen does not affect the severity of the pain in these patients."

"Why is that?"

"Because the smooth muscle spasm in the viscous organ creates pain independently of palpation—unlike peritoneal pain, which is associated with its own set of clinical conditions."

A slide with bright green lettering appeared. It said:

PERITONEAL PAIN SYNDROME: A CONSTANT, SEVERE, AND
GENERALIZED ABDOMINAL DISCOMFORT CAUSED BY
INFLAMMATION OF THE PERITONEAL WALL.

Lynne quickly proceeded to the next slide:

PERITONEAL PAIN: REBOUND TENDERNESS,
THE PHYSICAL HALLMARK

"You see how this condition is different?" Lynne asked. "Peritoneal pain is caused by irritation and inflammation of the peritoneal wall. Any number of inflammatory conditions can produce this. As you probably know, appendicitis is the most common. But there's also diverticulitis, ectopic pregnancy, and abdominal infection. In fact, any condition that causes hemorrhage into the peritoneum produces this syndrome. That's because blood is very irritating to the peritoneal tissue."

"Remember, the nature of peritoneal inflammation is such that patients are usually very still," explained Lynne. "They don't writhe on the stretcher. They like to remain as motionless as pos-

---

sible, because any shifting or stretching of the peritoneal wall causes excruciating pain. Coughing usually produces pain in patients with peritoneal inflammation, and you can ask the patient to cough as a diagnostic maneuver. So you see, peritoneal pain is quite different from colicky pain syndrome, and the underlying conditions are also different."

> If the patient has abdominal pain as a primary symptom and there is also vomiting, the 60-Second EMT should consider a bowel obstruction as a likely cause.

I could see the importance of recognizing the difference between colicky and peritoneal pain. Donnelly's division of abdominal pain into these two pathways was going to be a time-saver. As I thought about this the next slide appeared. It read:

VOMITING SYNDROMES

"Frequently, the patient with abdominal pain also has nausea and vomiting," Lynne explained. "As a rule, you have to be suspicious of the following conditions."

She flicked to the next slide:

CAUSES OF VOMITING SYNDROMES: PAIN, BOWEL OBSTRUCTION, GASTROENTERITIS, GALLSTONES, KIDNEY STONES, MYOCARDIAL INFARCTION, ELEVATED INTRACRANIAL PRESSURE.

"The key here," she said, "is to remember that vomiting is often a nonspecific symptom that's caused by something other than an abdominal condition. Myocardial infarction and intracerebral hemorrhage are two of the more serious causes. I think this slide makes that point. On the other hand, of course, if the patient has abdominal pain as a primary symptom and there is also vomiting, the 60-Second EMT should consider a bowel obstruction as a likely cause."

Lynne advanced the carousel, revealing the next slide.

HEMORRHAGIC SYNDROMES: PROVIDE ALS TRANSPORT, INSTITUTE MAXIMAL PRECAUTIONS, MONITOR BLOOD PRESSURE.

"It goes without saying that any patient who is vomiting bright red blood (hematemesis) or coffee-ground material, or has dark, tarry (melanotic) stools or bright red blood per rectum (hemato-chezia), needs aggressive therapy," Lynne pointed out.

"Jerry feels that any patient with a gastrointestinal hemorrhage, with or without pain, should be transported by an ALS unit to a medical facility expeditiously. If shock-like symptoms are present, start an IV and titrate to a systolic BP of 100. These patients can sink fast."

The next slide appeared.

UPPER GI BLEEDING	LOWER GI BLEEDING
GASTRIC ULCER	NEOPLASM
GASTRITIS	HEMORRHOIDS
PEPTIC ULCER	ANGIOMA
ESOPHAGEAL VARICES	DIVERTICULITIS

"When Donnelly encounters a patient who gives a history of bleeding from the GI tract," the instructor said, "he tries to ascertain in which of these categories the bleeding belongs." "Now look at this next slide—it's very important to consider this possibility in the assessment of young and middle-aged women with abdominal pain and hypotension, syncope, or weakness."

ECTOPIC PREGNANCY: SUSPECT THIS CONDITION IN A FEMALE PATIENT WITH ABDOMINAL PAIN WHEN ANY OF THE FOLLOWING ARE PRESENT: PALLOR, WEAKNESS, HYPOTENSION, SYNCOPE, SHOULDER PAIN, VAGINAL BLEEDING.

"This is one of the most important slides in the 60-Second Assessment of Abdominal Pain," Lynne emphasized. "Ectopic pregnancy can be a great masquerader."

"Why is that?" I asked.

"Because the sexual and menstrual history can lead the EMT astray," she said, flipping to the next slide:

WARNING! THE MENSTRUAL AND SEXUAL HISTORY ARE NOT ALWAYS RELIABLE IN PATIENTS WITH ECTOPIC PREGNANCY. TREAT PATIENT ON THE BASIS OF SYMPTOMS AND VITAL SIGNS.

"Can you give me an example of what you mean?" I asked.

"Sure," she said. "I remember the time Jerry and I were dispatched to see a 29-year-old secretary who had collapsed in front of the word processor at the law office where she worked. We arrived on the scene and discovered a young woman lying on the floor with a 95-systolic blood pressure. She was very pale, had a greenish-yellow look, and was extremely weak. I thought she was going to go out on us any second. With the little bit of strength she had left, she said, 'My belly hurts; I think I've got the stomach flu.'"

"What did you and Donnelly do?" I asked.

"Jerry leaned over to me, so the patient couldn't hear, and whispered, 'Lynne, this woman has an ectopic—we better work fast.'"

"He said that before even taking a history."

"That's right. You wanted to know why they call Jerry Donnelly the 60-Second EMT. Well, with young women who have abdominal pain and low BPs, you might say he's more like the 10-Second EMT. Jerry knew that an ectopic pregnancy is equal in severity to a shotgun blast to the abdomen. Before you could say 'stat', Jerry put in a large-bore IV line and started fluids wide open and applied a PASG. We loaded her onto the stretcher and headed, Code 3, for the hospital. En route, when her blood pressure finally climbed to 110 and she'd stabilized somewhat, he asked her some questions. She told us she had an IUD in place and there was no way she could be pregnant. She also said that her last menstrual period was 4 weeks ago and it was normal."

"I suppose Jerry had to rethink his assessment," I offered.

"Not at all. He explained that IUDs are associated with a higher-than-normal incidence of ectopic pregnancies and that in about half of the cases, patients with an ectopic don't give a history of having missed a period. He palpated her lower abdomen and she had rebound tenderness—peritoneal irritation because of hemorrhage."

"So what happened?"

"She had a positive pregnancy test in the emergency department and her pelvic ultrasound demonstrated bleeding from an ectopic pregnancy. The gynecologist whisked her to surgery and removed an ectopic pregnancy and, I might add, three units of blood from her abdomen."

"That's an instructive case," I admitted. "I don't think I'll ever miss an ectopic pregnancy again. By the way, I assume that because of the intra-abdominal hemorrhage, patients with ectopic pregnancy have peritoneal irritation syndrome."

"That's right," Lynne said. "Most of the time, they have abdominal rebound tenderness."

Lynne pushed the button on her remote unit and an unusual

slide appeared on the screen. Each letter was a different color and the two words on the slide were:

GUT PAINS

"Is that your parting shot?" I asked.

"Not quite," she said. "This is my pride and joy."

"Well, it is a beautiful slide," I assured her. "But GUT PAINS—your pride and joy? I don't get it."

"I better explain," Lynne said, quickly flashing a series of slides, each of which had a single letter plastered over the entire image. The letters spelled out "GUT PAINS."

"When Jerry and I reviewed the 60-Second Assessment of Abdominal Pain, we felt something was missing," she explained. "What our module didn't have was a simple mnemonic device for remembering, classifying, and sorting out all the important causes of abdominal pain that fell under the various syndromes I've been telling you about. Well, GUT PAINS is the solution to that problem. Let me take you through it."

My hostess projected eight more slides, each of them listing abdominal conditions associated with each of the letters. It was an elegant way to remember the variety of disorders that need to go through the mind of an EMT when he or she is assessing the patient with abdominal pain.

"*G* stands for gallbladder stones, gas pains, gastroenteritis, gastritis, and gynecologic emergencies," Lynne said proudly. "Isn't that simple?"

"Yeah, that's clever," I said. "Go on."

"Okay. The *U* in GUT PAINS stands for ulcer disease, both gas-

---

GUT PAINS

G for Gallbladder stones, Gas pains, Gastroenteritis, Gastritis, Gynecologic emergencies.
U for Ulcer disease.
T for Trauma-induced abdominal injury.
P for Pancreatitis, PID, and Pregnancy (ectopic).
A for Abdominal Aortic Aneurysm, Appendicitis, Alcoholic gastritis, and Angina.
I for Ischemia, Intestinal obstruction, and Infections.
N for Neoplasm.
S for Spasm of the esophagus and Splenic rupture.

tric and peptic," she explained. "The *T* represents trauma-induced abdominal injury. Most often, we're talking about splenic rupture. It also stands for twisting conditions such as volvulus or testicular torsion, which is seen in young men and, on occasion, can have referred abdominal pain as the principal symptom."

I could see I was going to like what the rest of the letters had to offer.

"The *P* stands for pancreatitis, perforated ulcer, pelvic inflammatory disease (PID), and pregnancy of the ectopic variety," said Lynne. "See, you can take these conditions and plug them into the abdominal pain syndromes. If you combine both approaches, the syndromes and the mnemonic, you have a comprehensive and systematic approach to assessing abdominal pain."

I could see from Lynne's enthusiasm that she was very proud of this component of the 60-Second Abdominal Exam. And I believed she had good reason to be. The next slide appeared.

"The *A* in GUT PAINS stands for some very important conditions," she explained. "Abdominal aortic aneurysm, appendicitis, alcoholic gastritis, and abdominal angina. The *I* is equally important. It stands for intestinal obstruction, ischemia of the bowel, and infections."

"I can't believe how complete this is," I approved.

"The *N* stands for neoplasm," she said, "which can cause either intestinal obstruction—a colicky syndrome; or bleeding—the hemorrhagic syndrome. That leaves *S*, which stands for spasm of the esophagus and splenic rupture—another reminder in trauma cases."

Lynne advanced to the next, and last, slide which read

ABDOMINAL PAIN: DEVELOP A GUT FEELING
FOR THIS URGENT CONDITION

Then she went back to the booth and turned on the light.

"That was quite a show," I said.

"Thanks, I'm glad you enjoyed it," Lynne responded. "As you can see, Jerry Donnelly's 60-Second Assessment of Abdominal Pain is a class act from beginning to end."

ABDOMINAL PAIN

I. It helps to think of abdominal complaints in terms of the presenting symptom complexes: Those producing **Back** pain; those with **Peritoneal** symptoms and signs; those producing **Colicky** pain and **Vomiting**; **Hemorrhagic** disorders; and **Gynecologic** problems with abdominal pain. The following represent key points to remember about these syndromes.

A. **Back Pain.** Every patient who complains of back pain, especially trauma patients and those over the age of 60 without a prior history of trauma or back problems, should have a quick examination of the abdomen. Make sure that palpation of the abdomen does not reproduce the patient's back pain. Following this process, you should be able to ascertain the following abdominal causes of back pain:

1. **Abdominal Aortic Aneurysm.** The patient with an abdominal aortic aneurysm may actually have sciatica (pain shooting down the leg from the back) from dissection of the aneurysm into the sciatic nerve. Additional features include a history of hypertension, lack of pulses in the legs, hypotension, and, rarely, an abdominal bruit.

2. **Cholelithiasis.** Gallstone pain sometimes occurs as isolated right-thoracic or interscapular pain. This pain usually occurs with nausea and 1 to 2 hours after meals. Palpation of the right upper quadrant will produce the same back pain.

3. **Pancreatitis.** Most frequently associated with alcoholism or trauma, pancreatitis will often cause vomiting and hypovolemia. Patients sometimes will be hunched over and writhing, since movement does not make their pain worse; they cannot find a comfortable position.

4. **Perforated Ulcer.** Back pain from perforated ulcer is usually associated with **Peritoneal** signs and symptoms (see "Peritoneal Pain" below). However, with a posterior penetration into the

lesser peritoneal sac, back pain may be the only symptom.

B. **Colicky Pain.** By definition, colicky pain is spasmodic and therefore, waxes and wanes over time. It usually results from the spasm of the smooth muscle of the visceral organs trying to overcome an obstruction. The following are important causes of obstruction and colicky abdominal pain:

   1. **Bowel Obstruction** is associated with persistent vomiting and the absence of bowel movements and with gas, hypovolemia, abdominal distension, and absent bowel sounds with occasional rushes.

   2. **Renal Obstruction.** Most often associated with kidney stones, renal obstruction pain occurs in the flanks, is very severe, frequently radiates into the groin or the testicles, and is often also associated with vomiting.

   3. **Gallbladder Obstruction.** See previous section under "Back Pain."

C. **Peritoneal Pain.** The hallmark of peritoneal pain is the presence of "guarding"—producing a rigid, board-like abdomen and rebound tenderness (see text). This results from irritation of the peritoneum from blood (e.g., ruptured spleen), contents from any ruptured organ (e.g., perforated ulcer), or primary infection.

   1. Patients with peritoneal pain will be lying very still, since any movement, such as being transferred to your ambulance, will markedly worsen their pain.

   2. They also will have very quiet to absent bowel sounds (without rushes).

D. **Vomiting Syndromes.** Remember that vomiting is a very nonspecific syndrome and can be caused by a wide variety of diseases. In addition to the previously mentioned syndromes of bowel obstruction, gallstones, and kidney stones, the following can also produce a vomiting syndrome:

   1. **Pain** from any cause can cause vomiting in sus-

ceptible patients. This, of course, must be a diagnosis of exclusion.

2. **Myocardial Infarction**, as described in the chestpain and geriatric-emergencies modules.
3. **Elevated Intracranial Pressure.**

E. **Hemorrhagic Syndromes.** Distinguish these into *upper* and *lower* GI bleeding sources. The reason for doing so is that upper GI bleeding will often result in hemodynamic compromise (hypovolemia, shock), whereas lower GI bleeding most often will not.

1. **Upper GI.** The hallmarks of upper GI syndrome include a previous history of peptic ulcer disease (epigastric pain *relieved* by food ingestion: duodenal ulcer; pain *worsened* by food ingestion while swallowing: esophageal; or pain 5 to 30 minutes after ingestion: gastric); the ingestion of substances corrosive to the gastric lining (aspirin, alcohol, anti-inflammatory agents). Bleeding from esophageal varices occurs in patients with a history of cirrhosis.

   a. Blood originating from the esophagus to the mid-small intestine will turn the stool black (called melena). If the UGI bleeding is brisk, the stool will appear maroon.

   b. Vomited blood originating from the upper GI tract will look red to maroon. If not brisk, it will turn black (because of reaction with the stomach's acid) and appear in small clumps, and the vomitus will resemble coffee grounds.

2. **Lower GI.** Patients with lower GI bleeding frequently have crampy lower abdominal pain that is relieved by bowel movements. The bowel movements are usually bright red in appearance. REMEMBER: Bright red lower blood coming from the rectum may actually be coming from a massive upper GI hemorrhage. Lower GI hemorrhages, however, usually do not bleed appreciably and do not often produce hemodynamic impairment.

F. **Gynecologic Syndromes.** *Think ectopic!* **Ectopic pregnancy** is of extreme urgency and should be the diagnosis until proven otherwise in all women of child-bearing age (≤50 y/o) who have any of the following symptoms:
   1. Lower abdominal pain.
   2. Hypotension.
   3. Shoulder-tip pain with abdominal pain.
   4. Vaginal bleeding.
   5. Syncope.

II. Remember **GUT PAINS**:
   G for Gallbladder stones, Gas pains, Gastroenteritis, Gastritis, Gynecologic emergencies.
   U for Ulcer disease.
   T for Trauma-induced abdominal injury.
   P for Pancreatitis, PID, and Pregnancy (ectopic).
   A for Abdominal Aortic Aneurysm, Appendicitis, Alcoholic gastritis, and Angina.
   I for Ischemia, Intestinal obstruction, and Infections.
   N for Neoplasm.
   S for Spasm of the esophagus and Splenic rupture.

III. 60-Second Triage:
   A. **ALS:**
      1. Any back pain in elderly patients with no prior history of trauma or of previous back pain—especially if associated with orthostatic hypotension, history of hypertension, and/or unequal or absent pulses in the lower extremities.
      2. All patients with peritoneal signs.
      3. Any abdominal pain with hemodynamic compromise (including orthostatic hypotension).
      4. Patients with colicky pain consistent with intestinal obstruction.
      5. Any elderly patient with nausea and vomiting of uncertain etiology.
      6. Upper GI hemorrhage.
   B. **BLS:**
      Most patients not in the above-mentioned syndromes.

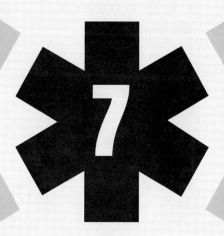

The 60-Second Assessment of the HIV-Positive Patient

arranged to meet Lisa Stone after her inservice session on AZT prophylaxis in needle-stick injuries. Her current interest was in reducing risk of AIDS transmission following exposure. She and Jerry had worked together on prehospital teaching of AIDS emergencies. Her work with Jerry on body substance isolation (BSI) and universal precautions reduced his unit's blood exposure to almost zero.

Prehospital care providers participate in delivery of medical care to HIV-positive and AIDS patients regardless of the setting they practice in.

Lisa had worked in the Emergency Department for over 15 years and, with her experience and skills, had developed an education program for the department. She and Jerry had discussed problems that providers have in understanding the subtleties of managing AIDS emergencies and in addressing concerns of personal risk.

After meeting in her office and taking a minute to admire her awards for clinical and teaching skills, we got down to business.

"Did you know current estimates of HIV infection and AIDS prevalence are now in the range of 1 for every 250 individuals in this country?" she began. "And you probably already know the 'classic' high risk groups: homosexuals, bisexuals, those with multiple sexual partners, and intravenous drug abusers who share needles. But did you know the HIV virus has also spread to those who are not in these high-risk groups? This means that prehospital care providers participate in delivery of medical care to HIV-positive and AIDS patients regardless of the setting they practice in." Lisa added that the number of people infected was still increasing.

"We're all concerned about the risk of acquiring AIDS through accidental exposure to known AIDS patients," I said, "but if the history of AIDS is not available or is unknown to the patient, adequate protection may not be taken. Add to that the fact that up to 15% of emergency transports involve patients who are HIV positive and you have one very scary scenario on your hands."

Up to 15% of emergency transports involve patients who are HIV-positive.

"You're absolutely right," said Lisa, "which emphasizes the need for BSI and universal precautions on all calls! Since all patients should be considered risks for transmitting HIV infection,

Protect Yourself

Use these precautions on *all* calls:

1. Discard sharps and never recap.
2. Manage the scene as much as possible.
3. Use gloves for all blood or fluid contact.
4. Wear eye protection.
5. Use gloves for cleaning soiled objects and surfaces.
6. No mouth-to-mouth respirations.
7. Cover any open skin lesions on your hands or body.

EMTs must use universal procedures and BSI procedures to (1) Discard sharps and never recap, (2) Use scene management as much as possible because there is less risk to the medical personnel in a controlled situation, (3) Use gloves for all blood or fluid contact, (4) Wear eye protection, (5) Use gloves for cleaning or discarding any soiled object, (6) Engage in no mouth-to-mouth respirations, and, finally, (7) Cover any open skin lesions on your hands or body when working."

"Those sound like basic precautions that would be easy to remember."

How simple, I thought. Protect yourself from needle stick by discarding sharps instead of recapping needles, and be extra careful when dealing with any blood and body fluids. Wearing gloves and eye protection and using a bag valve-mask instead of mouth-to-mouth resuscitation would take care of that. She's right, too, about maintaining control at the scene—less chance of accidents occurring that way.

Lisa began again, "It's important to realize that the same health problems that are seen in the general population also affect HIV patients. Nevertheless, patterns do exist for many diseases. Altered level of consciousness (ALOC) is a common complaint for the AIDS patient.

Altered level of consciousness (ALOC) is a common complaint for the AIDS patient.

"Standard therapy—thiamine, D5W, and Narcan—is given as part of the ALOC protocol, but there are further considerations. History should be obtained as best as possible. Because of altered level of consciousness, the patient may not be able to give an accurate history, so any available history from bystanders at the scene should be obtained. Remember, though, that bystanders, friends, and relatives may be reluctant to give you an accurate history."

She continued, "Meningitis is a very common complication of AIDS. Deficient immune system function predisposes not only to the typical meningitis infections, but also to a variety of unusual bacterial, fungal, parasitic, and viral pathogens." I thought of the cases of meningitis I had seen. The patients all had appeared very ill with a high fever and terrible headache. Several that had turned out to have pneumococcal meningitis were lethargic to nearly comatose.

"High fever, reports of severe headache, and nuchal rigidity require stabilization with oxygen, IV fluids, and rapid transport since bacterial meningitis would be a major concern. However, the presentation for AIDS patients is often much more subtle. We have a patient in the hospital now that Jerry saw last week. As I remember, he was called to a restaurant for a 28-year-old male who was very agitated. Jerry's partner took vital signs, which showed a tachycardia at 110 but were otherwise normal. Jerry asked for a history from the patient's friend, who said that he had had a mild headache intermittently for about a week and increasingly bizarre behavior. He had not complained of any fever, and she knew of no trauma. Jerry asked about medications and illness and found that the patient had tested HIV positive but had not had any illness related to this and was not on medication. He had no evidence of head trauma and had a normal neck and neurologic exam. His friend added that he had experienced very strange thoughts, and she suggested that Jerry transport them to a psychiatric setting. That seemed a reasonable request since the man really seemed not to have a physical cause for his agitation. Because of his history of HIV infection, Jerry transported him to a full-service emergency department, where a head CT revealed multiple calcific nodules, and spinal fluid analysis ultimately revealed a toxoplasmosis infection. Mild headache, apparently psychotic behavior, and confusion can all be subtle presentations of meningitis even though the usual findings for meningitis are absent."

Mild headache, apparently psychotic behavior, and confusion can all be subtle presentations of meningitis even though the usual findings for meningitis are absent.

"Because of CNS infections, seizures can result as a complication. Again, the patient may not have seemed ill before the seizure occurred. Seizures, especially first-time, are dramatic enough usually to initiate emergency aid. If they are witnessed, a characteristic description may be obtained. If the patient

---

The 4 "Ms" for Altered Levels of Consciousness in AIDS Patients

Meningitis	Medication
Malnutrition	Missing Oxygen (Hypoxia)

---

is found unresponsive, or still has postictal immobility, a description of the seizure may be given by whoever initiated the call. AIDS patients are at risk for seizures from the same causes as the general population—head trauma, alcohol withdrawal, strokes, or CNS trauma, etc. However, CNS abscesses, viral encephalitis, and infections such as cryptococcus or toxoplasmosis cause tissue reaction or mass lesions in the brain and can precipitate seizures. When the level of consciousness is altered, always consider the basics as well as the more complicated possibilities.

Gastrointestinal infections and fever are common in AIDS patients.

There are four "Ms" that explain ALOC in patients with AIDS. Meningitis is the first consideration of ALOC. The second 'M' is malnutrition. Food intake may be poor because of nausea, debilitating effects of AIDS, and fluid and electrolyte loss from illness. The third 'M' is medication. This can be overdose or side effects of prescribed therapy. The fourth 'M' is hypoxia."

"How can you get 'M' from hypoxia?" I asked. "By 'M'issing oxygen," Lisa replied with a smile. "Pulmonary infiltrates are also a common affliction of AIDS patients, and profound hypoxia may result.

"Gastrointestinal infections with fever from chronic bacterial and parasitic infections are common in AIDS patients. Combine fluid loss from diarrhea, chronic fever, and poor appetite with electrolyte deficiencies, and altered mental status becomes a common problem."

Lisa continued, "Assess skin texture, turgor, and the mucous membranes. If the patient is able to sit up or stand, check orthostatic blood pressure and begin aggressive fluid therapy if needed. Malnutrition refers to fluids as well as nutrients and electrolytes.

"When faced with the diagnosis of a terminal illness, deterioration of health and functioning, potential ostracism from society, depression, and suicidal ideation can follow."

I thought how I would react to being told I had a fatal, incurable illness, and this made sense.

Lisa's tone remained serious. "In assessing altered level of consciousness, a suicide attempt must be considered. If a history can be obtained of a possible ingestion of drugs or poison, careful data gathering is important. This would entail the same assessment that Jerry uses for toxicological emergencies.

> The same infections that affect the general populace can affect AIDS patients but other more unusual infections occur.

"The therapy of AIDS and AIDS complications is complex, and not all physicians are familiar with specific drug treatments. Having the names of medications written down or bottles available can be crucial to emergency care. Many drugs are experimental and are only available outside of the country. A network exists to bring these drugs into the United States. Pills taken may never have been prescribed, so no hospital records will be available.

"Again," Lisa emphasized, "the same infections that affect the general populace can affect AIDS patients but other more unusual infections occur. Pneumocystis pneumonia has a very high prevalence among AIDS patients and can be a very subtle presentation."

"Can you give me an example?" I asked.

"Sure. Jerry's assessment of a patient brought in last week is a good one. He was called to the scene by family members for a 24-year-old male who was short of breath. When Jerry arrived, the young man was sitting on the couch apparently comfortable and talking and in no respiratory distress. Jerry noted a resting respiratory rate of 28, however. After walking across the room the patient became more tachypneic, and Jerry noticed a slight bluish tint to his lips. He took further history and found that the man had had a dry cough and some weakness for several days. On exam, auscultation of his lungs revealed them to be almost completely clear. But a portable SaO_2 monitor showed an O_2 saturation of 81%. Jerry established supplemental oxygen and transported the patient to the emergency department for further evaluation. A chest x-ray revealed extensive infiltrate throughout both lung fields, and ABGs showed arterial oxygen of 41% of room air. This was a classic case of pneumocystis pneumonia. Very minimal finding and profound hypoxia . . . 'missing oxygen'!"

I had recently seen two cases of tuberculosis in young patients and asked about this and my risk of acquiring TB.

"That's a real concern," replied Lisa. "Tuberculosis is making

Signs and Symptoms of Tuberculosis

Cough	Weakness
Hemoptysis	Weight loss
Fever	Fatigue
Shortness of Breath	Positive PPD Test

a resurgence. Productive cough and hemoptysis in the AIDS patient will always require further evaluation. The patient and EMT should both be masked for protection against possible mucous membrane exposure. Classic presentation includes cough, hemoptysis, fever, and shortness of breath. The patient may also give a history of weakness, weight loss, fatigue, and a positive PPD test. Tuberculosis is difficult to treat, at best, and resistant strains are emerging.

"We all are concerned about the risk of acquiring AIDS through accidental exposure to known AIDS patients. Presentations such as altered level of consciousness, obtundation, seizure, fever, and dehydration are fairly routine and common in calls, and they represent high risk of HIV infection. Unfortunately, if the history of AIDS is not available or is unknown to the patient, adequate precautions for protection may not be taken. Hence the need for universal precautions and BSI. All patients are a risk for transmitting HIV infection. Precautions include: (1) Discarding sharps, never recapping; (2) scene management as much as possible, because there is less risk to medical personnel in a controlled situation; (3) gloves for all blood or fluid contact; (4) eye, nose, and mouth protection; (5) gloves for cleaning or discarding any soiled object; (6) no mouth-to-mouth respirations; and (7) not working with any exposed open skin lesions."

Lisa finished and said, "I gave you the precautions twice because I want you to remember them."

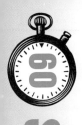

HIV-Positive Patient

1. **Body Substance Isolation (BSI) and Universal Precautions.** Up to 15% of transports involve HIV infection. Even if HIV is not the problem, BSI and universal protections protect you from other communicable diseases.
2. AIDS patients are susceptible to the same illnesses as the general public.
3. Four "Ms" in altered level of consciousness:
   a. Meningitis, frequently atypical.
   b. Malnutrition, fluid and electrolyte deficiency.
   c. Medication, overdosage, and unusual drugs.
   d. Missing oxygen, severe hypoxia with minimal lung findings.
4. Do not let your emotions or personal feelings cloud the issue. HIV-positive and AIDS patients are indeed that—*patients.* Afford them the same level of care you would expect for yourself.

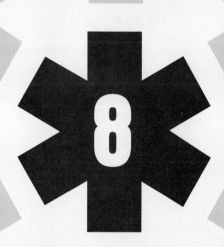

The 60-Second
Multiple Trauma
Assessment

o use an old expression, Jeff Clark had seen it all: the bad and the good—actually, much more of the former than the latter. As a Green Beret medic in Vietnam, Clark had transported more than 1500 critically injured soldiers from the battlefield to military hospitals outside the combat zone. Most of the injured required urgent intervention, fast decision-making, and aggressive therapy; Clark, Donnelly told me, had a reputation for never buckling in the call of duty. "If you were shot through the chest or abdomen while doing combat in Nam," Donnelly said, "Jeff Clark was the guy you'd want stabilizing you in the field."

Clark returned from the war with a Congressional Medal of Honor, two Purple Hearts, and a vast arsenal of useful skills. The problem was that he was in no psychological shape to use them. Clark's adjustment to normal life was a stormy one. He was diagnosed as suffering from post-traumatic stress disorder; and for about two years after the war ended, he endured long periods of depression, horrifying flashbacks of grisly combat experiences, and general irritability. He spent much of his time working at odd jobs and playing the keyboard for a local band.

According to Donnelly, after six months of intensive counseling Clark's outlook on life began to brighten. At his counselor's urging, he volunteered at a local emergency department, where physicians, nurses, and EMTs quickly recognized him as a shining star in assessing and managing patients who had sustained severe trauma. In fact, it was in the emergency department that Donnelly and Clark first met and discussed the possibility of developing a 60-second exam for multiple trauma victims.

The two men focused their attention initially on a new disaster management program for the community. Donnelly drew on Clark's experience in Vietnam to develop protocols for the new system. It was soon rated one of the finest in the country. Although Donnelly had become a proponent of an "enlightened scoop-and-run and treat en route" policy for multiple trauma, he also recognized the importance of refining assessment and critical intervention protocols for patients with life-threatening injuries. This led to the development of The 60-Second Multiple Trauma Exam, in which Clark played a critical role. My purpose in visiting Clark was to find out what they had come up with.

The day I met Jeff Clark, he had just finished a long day of EMT testing. He had overseen the multiple trauma section of the exam and, judging from the look on his face, was a little frustrated by the performance of the EMTs he had just tested.

"You look worn out," I said as we shook hands.

"I am," Jeff sighed. "You know, I've tested 28 EMTs and every one of them should have passed the multiple trauma section of the paramedic exam. But many did not, and that makes me a little discouraged."

"Why?" I asked.

"Because on a skill-by-skill basis, all of the people I tested should have passed."

"So what's the problem?" I asked.

"The problem is, many of the EMTs didn't have an overall plan for initial assessment and management of trauma patients. Before the exam was over, most of them started IV lines and managed the airway. But I wasn't satisfied with the sequence and aggressiveness of their approach with patients who were clearly in shock and needed emergency intervention."

"So what's your solution?"

"My suggestion is that they learn the protocols and guidelines offered by Jerry Donnelly's 60-Second Multiple Trauma Assessment. If they get those principles under their belt, they'll sail right through the EMT exam," Jeff said confidently.

"In what ways does the 60-second assessment speed up reaction time?" I asked.

"For one thing, the approach emphasizes aggressive treatment of the patient," Clark informed me. "If you are on your way to a bad motor vehicle accident or to a victim with a gunshot wound to the chest, you have to start thinking immediately about treating shock—even before you get there."

"You mean be prepared for the worst," I said.

"That's right," Clark agreed, "because except for tension pneumothorax or cardiac arrhythmias, the only way you are going to lose a multiple trauma patient is by not being aggressive with airway management, C-spine stabilization, and IV access (usually during transport). On the way to the scene, the 60-Second EMT will already be thinking about basic airway management with C-spine stabilization, ventilatory assistance, and ET intubation."

> If you are on your way to a bad motor vehicle accident or to a victim with a gunshot wound to the chest, you have to start thinking immediately about treating shock—even before you get there.

"But doesn't every EMT think of these things?" I inquired.

"Eventually they do," said Clark, "but the key is to know, within the time frame of the Golden Minute, that these maneuvers are going to be required and be able to implement them sooner rather than later. That's what frustrated me about the EMTs I tested today. They weren't systematic about assessment. They required too much information before initiating management."

"Why do you think that is?"

"I think it's because they're not primed to intervene aggressively on the basis of limited information."

"What do you mean by that? Can you be more specific?"

"Sure. For example, the amount of information needed to start management for a critically traumatized patient is minimal. A rapid pulse and shallow respirations provide enough data to let you know the patient needs aggressive airway management, including lung ventilation with 100% O_2 and, possibly, intubation. If the patient is cyanotic or has a respiratory rate of less than 12 or a flail chest, the 60-Second EMT knows that intubation will be almost mandatory. All the paramedics who've seen Donnelly manage trauma patients remark about how quickly he moves once the vital signs have been obtained."

"Really?"

Jeff nodded. "Once he obtains the vital signs, he's programmed to recheck them to see whether his therapy is working. For a patient in critical condition, only pulse and respiration are mandatory."

"This assessment seems somewhat superficial to me," I remarked.

"It may seem that way but the 60-Second EMT knows that most multiple trauma patients will deteriorate from one of six causes: Cardiac arrhythmias caused by metabolic acidosis, C-spine instability, Airway problems, Tension pneumothorax, Hemorrhagic blood loss, and Sucking chest wound. In fact, the 60-Second Multiple Trauma Assessment is based on the mnemonic that Jerry came up with called **CATHS**."

I thought about what Clark was saying and it seemed to make a lot of sense. Performing critical intervention and appropriate transport are the critical steps in managing trauma patients. The CATHS approach would efficiently orient an EMT toward the most likely causes of deterioration in multiple trauma victims, focusing clearly on the six types of organ failure that should be managed in the field.

"Does the primary survey provide enough information to treat the CATHS conditions?" I asked.

"Of course, or it wouldn't be useful," Jeff explained. "Let's go through CATHS and I'll explain how Jerry does it."

"Can you illustrate this approach using a case you and Jerry treated together?"

"No problem," he said. "I am thinking about a Sunday when we were called to the scene of a high-speed motorcycle accident. The dispatcher told us the driver wasn't wearing a helmet. En route to the scene, Jerry was already thinking about the possibility of a head injury."

"That makes sense," I interjected.

"Donnelly knew that head injuries not only require the obvious C-spine precautions, but aggressive airway management. Respiratory distress—usually on the basis of ataxic breathing or apnea—is the most common way that paramedics lose patients with head injury. So I guess Jerry was psyching himself up to intubate the patient if necessary. Anyway, we arrived at the scene and saw the victim lying on the road about 15 feet from the cycle."

"I guess that sight and knowing the mechanism of injury tipped you off immediately to the reality that you had a critically injured patient," I remarked.

"You're right. The 60-Second Trauma Exam emphasizes that point. Even before examining the patient, the 60-Second EMT will deduce, on the basis of the mechanism of injury alone, that aggressive intervention is going to be needed. That's why Jerry includes mechanism of injury as part of the 60-second evaluation. It's a powerful predictive instrument. In fact, it's not uncommon for Jerry to therapeutically intervene on the basis of mechanism of injury alone."

> Respiratory distress—usually on the basis of ataxic breathing or apnea—is the most common way that paramedics lose patients with head injury.

"What kind of shape was the patient in?"

"In pretty bad shape, not surprisingly," Jeff continued. "He was comatose, for one thing. His heart rate was 126 and irregular, respiratory rate 16 and labored, and systolic blood pressure was 80 palpable. On initial inspection we found a large laceration over the temporal area and an open chest wound with paradoxical movement of the left side of the chest. Breath sounds were present bilaterally and there was peripheral cyanosis."

"So did Jerry move down the CATHS pathway?" I asked.

"Not only that, he moved down the FAST CATHS pathway," Jeff informed me.

"FAST? As in 'Fast Action Saves Time'?"

"Absolutely! Multiple trauma is not the time for the CHOR, or Contemplative, History-Oriented approach. In this setting, it's FAST CATHS all the way."

I remembered reading about the fast pathway in Donnelly's Golden Minute. I thought it was neat the way he had combined the two mnemonics into "FAST CATHS."

Jeff continued. "Now let me show you how Jerry plugged his vital signs into the CATHS approach. On the basis of the low blood pressure, Jerry knew the patient was in shock and probably had severe internal hemorrhage and volume depletion. So he treated the *H* in CATH—hemorrhage—with bleeding control, large-bore IVs, and a fluid challenge."

"How much fluid did he give?"

"Since Jerry is familiar with some of the new theories on trauma management, he chose to limit the initial fluid bolus to 1000 ml. Jerry rarely gives over 2000 ml in the field without medical direction."

"Why the irregular pulse in such a young patient?" I asked.

"Good question. The irregular pulse worried both of us, and when we put him on the monitor, we noted PVCs. Jerry reasoned that the patient was severely acidotic on the basis of shock and hypoventilation and that the PVCs might be caused by cardiac irritability, the *C* in CATH. So he pushed some fluids to treat the hypoperfusion, and the cardiac arrhythmia improved. The peripheral cyanosis, flail chest, coma, and respiratory distress suggested the need for aggressive airway management. Jerry inserted a nasotracheal tube after C-spine stabilization. That took care of the *A* in CATH. The sucking chest wound was sealed and the flail chest was taped. That was the *S*. By the time Jerry and I had instituted the FAST CATHS therapies, his blood pressure had come up to 100 and his skin color had improved dramatically."

"What about the *T*, tension pneumothorax?" I inquired.

"Well, I'm glad you asked," Jeff said. "Because the *T* did eventually come into play. On the way to the hospital, ventilation became difficult, his blood pressure bottomed out, he lost his breath sounds on the right, and breath sounds on the left decreased. Unsealing the chest dressing did not improve conditions so Jerry performed a needle decompression of the right chest."

"What happened?"

"The air gushed out and we had a salvageable patient again," Jeff said with enthusiasm.

I had been treating trauma victims for a long time and could never fully grasp how to assess victims quickly enough to institute lifesaving therapies in time. Donnelly's FAST CATHS system did not cover all the other interventions required, such as those for extremity injuries, evisceration, and external bleeding. More important, however, it did cover the six conditions—cardiac arrhythmias, C-spine stabilization, airway problems, tension pneumothorax, hemorrhage, and sucking chest wounds—that made the difference between bringing a patient to the emergency department dead or alive.

Get the FAST CATHS system down and you will be a 60-Second EMT in no time.

"Thanks for taking the time to talk with me, Jeff," I said.

"You're welcome," he answered. "Get the FAST CATHS system down and you will be a 60-Second EMT in no time."

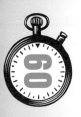

MULTIPLE TRAUMA

I. Time is of the essence. A general rule for the prehospital care of trauma is that **no intervention inessential for the maintenance of life should be done in the field, because time is more important.**
   A. Only the primary assessment (ABCs with C-spine stabilization) and resuscitation (see **FAST CATHS**) should be done in the field. All secondary surveys and procedures should be carried out in the ambulance en route to the hospital.
   B. The on-scene time should not exceed 10 minutes after extrication has been accomplished.
   C. Blood pressures should not be taken in the primary assessment. Blood pressures can be estimated in the primary assessment by the presence of various pulses:
      1. If the radial pulse is palpable, the systolic pressure will be above 88 mm Hg.
      2. If the femoral or carotid pulse is palpable, the systolic pressure will be above 70 and 60 mm Hg respectively.
II. Be prepared to intervene aggressively on the basis of limited information. For the critically injured trauma patient, assessment and treatment must proceed simultaneously.
   A. If the pulse is rapid, the patient will probably need IV access and volume replacement. Limit volume replacement to 2000 ml unless the base station physician directs otherwise. Some physicians feel that increasing BP or giving much volume may increase mortality
   B. Indications for intubation (**Note:** Any airway maneuver should only be done with manual stabilization of the neck and cricoid pressure):
      1. Apnea.
      2. Extensive flail chest.
      3. Facial or laryngeal trauma with no airway (cricothyroidotomy).

4. If the patient has marginally adequate ventilation (e.g., respiratory rate <12/min or >30-35/min) and is either comatose, in shock, or has an underlying pulmonary problem.

For patients with suspected increased intracranial pressure, trismus, or partial gag reflex, consider use of a "rapid sequence intubation" technique.

   C. PASG is controversial in prehospital care. It is definitely contraindicated in patients with pulmonary edema or with severe trauma above the diaphragm. Use in abdominal injuries, pelvic fracture, and long-bone fracture is still acceptable but controversial. Consult local protocols and medical command on the use of PASG.

III. Use **FAST CATHS** to anticipate critical problems in the trauma patient. **F**ast **A**ction **S**aves **T**ime for:
   Cardiac arrhythmias and **C**-spine instability.
   Airway problems.
   Tension pneumothorax.
   Hemorrhagic blood loss.
   Sucking chest wounds.

IV. Anticipate major trauma by the mechanism of injury:
   A. Penetrating injury to chest, abdomen, head, neck, and groin. **Note:** Never assume that there is only one penetrating wound. Always search for additional wounds, especially of the above listed areas.
   B. Falls of 20 feet or more.
   C. Automobile accidents in which:
      1. The differential velocities are 25 mph.
      2. There is rearward displacement of the front axle.
      3. There is rearward displacement of the front of the car by 20 inches.
      4. Passenger compartment intrusion, especially of 1 foot or more.
      5. Ejection of the patient.
      6. Rollover of the vehicle.
      7. Death of an occupant in the same vehicle.
      8. Pedestrian accidents.

V. **60-Second Triage:**
  A. **ALS**
    1. Any of the above-listed mechanisms of injury.
    2. Glasgow Coma Scale <13.
    3. Systolic blood pressure <90.
    4. Respiratory rate <10 or >29.
    5. Flail chest.
    6. Burns of >20% (adults) or 10% (children and geriatric patients) or those of the face or airway.
  B. **BLS:** Any trauma not included in the ALS criteria.

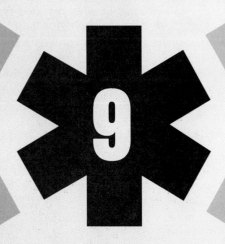

9

The 60-Second
Coma Exam

had heard many good things about Frank Zimmer. He had an admirable reputation and had been a keynote speaker at Donnelly's annual conference on the 60-Second EMT. A number of emergency physicians I had talked to considered him one of the outstanding EMTs in the community. His lecture entitled "The Prehospital Assessment and Management of Coma" was one of the best I had heard at an EMT conference.

Put simply, Frank Zimmer was smart. Only later did I learn that many of Frank's "pearls" about the prehospital assessment and management of coma had evolved during his tenure with Jerry Donnelly. For two years, they had been partners at the same base station hospital. Although Donnelly had moved on, they still kept in close touch. I predicted that Zimmer would be able add to my understanding of the Donnelly legend.

When I arrived at Frank's hospital, he was giving a group of elementary school children a guided tour through his rig. I stood back for a moment and watched. There were about twenty kids, and they all seemed intrigued by the life support equipment carried on each unit. Wide-eyed and chattering, they prowled through the ambulance as if they were in Disneyland. After several minutes, the kids were still asking questions about the cardiac monitor, the oxygen tank, and medications. Frank, who seemed to be enjoying the fuss, was very patient and answered all their questions. After a half-hour or so, their teacher finally pried them out of the ambulance and ushered them back into the hospital to continue their tour.

After the children left, I approached Zimmer.

"Hello," I said.

"Good to see you," Zimmer said, grabbing my hand and giving it a warm shake. "It's my day off, but I came in today to show these kids some of our equipment. It seemed they were interested in knowing what role EMTs play in the emergency medical system."

"That's great," I said.

"I know you're here to talk about Donnelly," Zimmer said with a smile. "I'm not surprised. I can't believe someone hasn't looked into this guy before. He's a very special person. And so is his 60-Second EMT Program."

"That's why I'm here," I confirmed.

Frank and I walked over to the soft drink machine and each bought a soda. He popped open his can, downed some cola, then launched into a discussion of the general principles underlying Donnelly's 60-Second Approach to Coma Assessment.

"Donnelly is as fast as they come, but he's also incredibly disciplined," Frank began. "There's a method to his 60-second madness. It's one thing to have a fund of knowledge. It's another thing to know exactly how to use it. Jerry has both bases covered."

"How so?" I inquired. I was trying to encourage Frank to give me some concrete examples of the 60-Second EMT in action. He did not disappoint me.

"I remember the time we were called to one of those fast-lane bars downtown," Zimmer continued. "Dispatch informed us there was an adolescent male unconscious in the downstairs rest room. The place was swarming with glossy-lipped teenagers. What a group. Wild clothes. Wild eyes. Several of the kids had iridescent hair spiked in every direction. The red-hot throb of punk rock music was filtering in from the club upstairs. It was a real scene. When we peeled away the layers in the crowd and finally got to the patient, we found a comatose teenager. He was barely breathing. One of his friends told us the victim had been drinking too much. There was no other history. At first I thought we were dealing with another teenager that couldn't hold his booze. We see a lot of that these days."

"Sounds like a logical first impression," I said.

"Well, I thought so too," Zimmer said, "but Jerry wasn't convinced that was the whole story.

" 'This guy is comatose,' he said. 'He's got pinpoint pupils. He's cyanotic. I think we may be dealing with a narcotic overdose. Let's institute the coma protocol, Stat!' "

"What happened next?" I inquired.

"Well, by this time the patient was almost apneic and I started bag-valve-mask ventilation," continued Zimmer. "Without wasting a second, Jerry started an IV and pushed 2 mg of Narcan®.

The 60-Second Coma Program calls for immediate implementation of the coma protocol regardless of what bystanders offer.

"Jerry said, 'I'm glad we got the IV quickly, but any time you can't you should give the Narcan IM or SL.'

"The patient's breathing and mental status improved within 30 seconds. When the kid was awake enough to give a history, he admitted that had shot up some heroin. Apparently, he hadn't told any of his friends what his drug habits were."

I had heard about so many cases in which bystanders had given histories that misled EMTs caring for comatose patients. It was refreshing to see that Donnelly's 60-Second Coma Program calls for immediate implementation of the coma protocol regardless of what bystanders offer.

"When you work on the streets, you can't take anything for granted," Frank explained. "Jerry likes to hammer away at that point. As he puts it, 'When you hear hoofbeats, you have to think first of horses.' In other words, the most common problems. But sometimes—and usually when you least expect it—those hoofbeats belong to zebras."

"What does Donnelly mean by 'zebras?' " I asked.

"He means the patient's problem is caused by something that catches you off guard, a condition that comes out of left field, something odd and unusual . . . a zebra," he answered.

I could see the importance of always being on your toes and looking out for the zebra, but I wasn't quite sure how the 60-Second EMT program protected the prehospital provider from the element of surprise.

"How does Donnelly cover his bases in situations like that?" I asked.

"With his 60-Second Coma Treatment Protocol," Frank said. "Maybe I can illustrate this point with a case. Jerry and I were working together one night and we were called to see a young female who had passed out in a nightclub. She was the lead singer in a hip-hop group called 'Yo Girls.'

"The place was a well-known hangout for drug dealers. When we got there, the girl was lying in the middle of the stage. She was barely responsive. Some of the kids who were huddled around her said they thought she had overdosed on something. At first glance, that seemed like the most logical explanation for her condition."

"So what did you do?"

"You mean what did Jerry do?" Frank grinned. "Within 20 seconds, he looked for obvious signs of trauma to the head and body; he smelled her breath for alcohol and ketones; he ran up and down her arms looking for needle marks; he looked for pinpoint pupils suggesting a narcotic overdose; and he probed her wrists and neck for medical alert tags."

"And?" I asked.

"Zilch!" Frank exclaimed. "Everything was negative. All we had was our primary survey, which revealed an unresponsive and diaphoretic patient. So the 60-second king started an IV, drew a tube of blood, and pushed some Narcan®. I expected her to wake up, but there was no response. I figured that she'd ingested something we couldn't reverse. I started bag-valve-mask ventilations and assumed we'd be loading her into the ambulance for transport. But then, without a moment's delay, Donnelly continued the coma protocol."

"You mean D_{50}?" I asked.

"Exactly!" he said. "Admittedly, it was a long shot, but he pushed 50 cc of $D_{50}W$ and her mental status improved dramatically. Within 30 seconds she was awake! I couldn't believe it."

"You mean it wasn't a drug overdose?"

"That's right," Frank smiled. "It was an insulin reaction. A bona fide 'zebra'—at least in that situation it was. We expected a drug overdose, not an insulin reaction. When the patient got her bearings back, she told us she was a diabetic and that her doctor had recently upped her insulin dosage. She told us she normally wore a medical alert bracelet but took it off when she was performing."

> Institute the three-drug coma protocol in *all* unresponsive patients, regardless of what the evidence at the scene suggests.

"I bet even the 60-Second EMT must have been a little surprised," I commented.

"He was," Frank admitted.

The fact was that Donnelly's handling of this case was impressive. His follow-through underscored the importance of instituting the three-drug coma protocol in *all* unresponsive patients, regardless of what the evidence at the scene suggests. Thiamine, 50% dextrose, and Narcan® rarely do any harm, and on occasion, you'll pick up that "zebra" and save a patient's life.

I thought it was time to share similar experiences I had had. "You know, Frank, it's amazing how many times I've seen EMTs bypass the coma protocol and miss a treatable condition."

"I've seen it, too," Frank confessed. "And it's a shame, because the drugs we use to treat coma in the field can't harm the patients. As Jerry and I spent more time working together, there were several other occasions when I saw patients recover from coma in situations I least expected."

"Do you remember any of those encounters?" I asked, deciding that I might as well pump him for all the information I could. From the little I had heard, Donnelly's 60-second "pitfalls" appeared to be almost as precious as his "pearls." I wanted to hear more about them.

Frank thought for a second and then said, "I'll never forget the time we were called to see a guy who was the driver in a single-car MVA. The windshield was cracked, and the man was unresponsive. We instituted our trauma procedure, stabilized the cervical spine, and placed the victim on a backboard.

"Just as we were about to transport, Jerry said, 'The guy probably has a head injury, but this is a single-car accident and he *is* comatose.'

"So I asked Jerry what he thought we should do," continued Frank. 'He's comatose,' Jerry repeated, 'which means there's an off chance that he may have passed out for some reason *before* impact. Let's give him the big three.' "

"The big three?" I queried.

"Yeah, you know: Thiamine, glucose, and Narcan®," Frank replied. "So Donnelly checked the patient's blood glucose with a Chemstrip, noted it was low, and then pushed some glucose. The guy woke up. I couldn't believe it. Here was another case of a diabetic with an insulin reaction in a situation that suggested some other cause for the patient's altered mental status. Instituting the coma protocol within the first minute of our encounter turned that case around."

The 60-second approach to the comatose victim relied heavily on the standard coma protocol. In one sense, it seemed so straightforward. I wasn't sure why Zimmer was stressing the point.

"Why is Donnelly so hung up on the importance of three-drug therapy in the 60-second approach?" I asked. "It seems like such an obvious point and such an easy treatment to implement."

> When a patient is comatose, do not try to be a diagnostic genius. Do not second-guess the patient. Just go ahead and use the coma protocol.

"It is!" Frank said. "And yet so many EMTs and paramedics still try to second-guess the situation and, in the process, forget—or exclude—the coma protocol. For this reason, Jerry's 60-second take-home lesson has always been: When a patient is comatose, do not try to be a diagnostic genius. Do not second-guess the patient. Just go ahead and use the coma protocol. Push the thiamine, glucose, and Narcan®. It won't harm the patient and he might get better when you least expect it."

I had to ask Frank if Jerry has ever addressed the controversy of giving glucose to a patient with a suspected increase in intracranial pressure, as in head injury. Frank said, "I asked Jerry about that.

"He told me, 'This matter is controversial. If you have Chemstrips, you can make an objective decision. If not, it becomes a judgment call.' If there is any chance of hypoglycemia, giving D_{50} is probably safer than withholding."

"And if they don't get better after the big three?" I asked.

"Then you implement Jerry's 60-second scheme for coma management," Frank said.

> The 60-second scheme for coma management is the ABCs.

"And what's that?"

"Above all, it's the ABCs," Frank explained. "Protect the airway, give moderate-flow O_2, monitor cardiac rhythm and blood pressure, and transport the patient in lateral recumbent position. Use an extrication collar and backboard with the patient supine if you suspect trauma. Always protect the patient from aspiration."

The 60-Second Coma Plan had a lot going for it. But I had also heard through the grapevine that, on occasion, Donnelly had given glucose to diabetic patients who were not comatose. I thought I would ask Frank about this.

I approached the issue gingerly. "Apparently, Donnelly has treated diabetics with IV glucose very early in their insulin reaction. In fact, I've heard he's pushed glucose in insulin-dependent diabetics whose sensorium was slightly clouded and in others who were confused and disoriented," I stated. "Is this really true?"

"As a matter of fact, it is," Frank informed me. "I've seen Jerry give glucose to known diabetics who were merely delirious, agitated, or who had slightly altered levels of consciousness. It's important to remember that, on many occasions, changes in mental status are the first, and most subtle, signs of impending coma. If hypoglycemia is responsible for the altered mental status, these patients will improve dramatically with glucose. Of course, if they are cooperative and have a gag reflex, he'll try oral glucose first."

> Remember that, on many occasions, changes in mental status are the first, and most subtle, signs of impending coma.

"It sounds as if he's really got a feel for these patients," I commented.

"Jerry has that sixth sense. No question about it," Zimmer confided. "Some of the paramedics around here think it's all instinct. Well, Jerry's got that all right, but he also knows his protocols to the letter. In my opinion, that's what separates him from the rest of the pack. The coma protocol is an important part of his 60-second approach. He tags it right on to the ABCs. Once he has assessed the patient's vital signs, he implements the coma protocol."

Signs and Symptoms of Hypoglycemia	
ADRENERGIC ACTIVATION	**DISTURBED CORTICAL FUNCTION**
Beta stimulation	Weakness
Tremulousness	Headache
Tachycardia	Blurred or double vision
Palpitations	Disturbed intellectual function
Diaphoresis	Amnesia
Faintness	Incoordination or paralysis
Anxiety	Seizures
Hunger	Coma
Gastric hypermotility	Brainstem dysfunction
Nausea	

"What about coma in the setting of head trauma?" I asked Zimmer. "Does the 60-Second EMT have an approach that works in those cases?"

"As a matter of fact, he does," Frank said with enthusiasm. "Jerry's 60-Second Coma Exam includes features that can be used to indicate the urgency of treating and transporting a patient with trauma-induced coma."

This was something I wanted to hear more about. Learning to detect severe head injuries can be difficult.

Frank continued, "Jerry and I were once called to see a 7-year-old boy who had run his bicycle into a car and hit his head on the pavement. When we arrived, we talked to bystanders who had seen the kid fall. They said he had been alert and talking just after impact. We examined the victim, who seemed alert and said he didn't want to go to the hospital. He had a nasty bump on his head over the temporal bone. I wasn't sure why Donnelly was moving so fast. But he was.

"Donnelly asked the child's mother if he had lost consciousness at any point after the fall.

"'Yes, it was sort of strange,' she said. 'Jimmy was fine right after hitting his head. In fact, he was talking and walking. Then, all of a sudden, he sort of went to sleep. He started to wake up again just before you arrived.'

"That's all Jerry needed to know. Once he had confirmed that the boy had had a period of lucidity and then become briefly unconscious, we gave high-flow O₂, immobilized the spine, and loaded that kid onto the rig. We transported him, Code 3, to the pediatric trauma center."

"Were you surprised?" I asked.

"Somewhat," Frank said. "I asked Jerry what the hurry was as we zig-zagged through rush-hour traffic with lights and siren. Jerry didn't mince his words.

" 'This kid is a set-up for an epidural hematoma,' he told me. 'It's classic, Frank. Right after head trauma, a patient's mental status may be fine, but then his level of consciousness starts to sink. This waxing and waning pattern is characteristic of an epidural. I think this kid's got a bleed in his head. He needs a neurosurgeon. And the sooner the better.' "

"Sounds like he was pretty confident about his assessment," I chimed in.

"That he was, but I've never heard him quite that panicked," Frank confided. "I'm sure everyone has told you that Jerry's usually so cool. Anyway, on the way to the hospital the boy's condition worsened. When we got there, the emergency physician sent him to CAT scan, Stat. The next thing we heard, the boy was in the operating room. He *did* have an epidural hematoma. If it weren't for Donnelly's judgment, the kid might not be alive today."

"So what's the key point in the 60-second assessment as it applies to head trauma?" I asked.

"The point that Jerry makes in his 60-second exam is that any patient with head trauma who has a period of lucidity after impact and then lapses into coma is a setup for an epidural hematoma. Especially if the injury is over the temporal area."

"Does the patient actually have to be completely comatose to require this degree of urgency?" I inquired.

"Absolutely not," Frank replied adamantly. "That's where a lot of EMTs get hung up. Patients can slip into coma rather quickly. It is very important to detect this high-risk group at once."

"What's the trick?" I asked.

"Well, Jerry likes to use key features of the Glasgow Coma Scale. The scale gives the 60-Second EMT a rough idea of how the patient is. In short, any impairment of consciousness, no matter how subtle, is an indication for vigilance and rapid transport."

> Any impairment of consciousness, no matter how subtle, is an indication for vigilance and rapid transport.

"What's the rush if the patient isn't comatose yet?" I asked.

"The patient can become comatose very quickly," Frank repeated. "That's why the 60-Second EMT has to look for signs of *impending* coma within the first minute of the encounter. And be prepared to take critical actions."

Glasgow Coma Scale

EYE OPENING		Total GCS Points
Spontaneous	4	14-15 = 5
To voice	3	11-13 = 4
To pain	2	8-10 = 3
None	1	5-7 = 2
		3-4 = 1
VERBAL RESPONSE		
Oriented	5	
Confused	4	
Inappropriate words	3	
Incomprehensible words	2	
None	1	
MOTOR RESPONSE		
Obeys command	6	
Localizes pain	5	
Withdrawn (pain)	4	
Flexion (pain)	3	
Extension (pain)	2	
None	1	
TOTAL TRAUMA SCORE		1-16

"Those signs are part of the Glasgow Coma Scale?" I queried.

"That's right," Frank continued. "Poor eye-opening responses, inappropriate or garbled speech, slow verbal responses, poor or absent motor activity, and abnormal flexion or extension are excellent indicators of neurologic impairment. They're part of the Glasgow scale. Amnesia, confusion, and sleepiness also indicate that you're dealing with a high-risk group."

> The 60-Second EMT has to look for signs of *impending* coma within the first minute of the encounter.

Frank stood up and walked back to the soda machine. I sat for a few moments reflecting on what I had just heard. The clarity of the 60-Second EMT approach to coma was one of its greatest assets. Frank made it clear that the 60-Second EMT had a host of clinical indicators that allowed him to discriminate between urgent and non-urgent neurosurgical cases and to detect high-risk groups that could deteriorate into coma very rapidly. He was also disciplined enough to use the coma protocol in every situation that called for it.

Frank Zimmer returned, sat down, and summarized what made Donnelly's 60-Second EMT approach to coma unique.

60-Second Management Algorithm For Patients With Coma

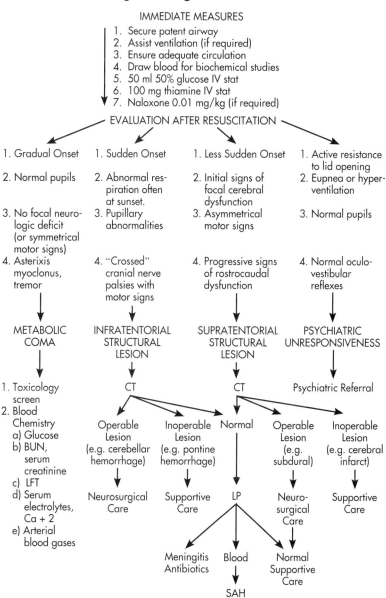

IMMEDIATE MEASURES
1. Secure patent airway
2. Assist ventilation (if required)
3. Ensure adequate circulation
4. Draw blood for biochemical studies
5. 50 ml 50% glucose IV stat
6. 100 mg thiamine IV stat
7. Naloxone 0.01 mg/kg (if required)

EVALUATION AFTER RESUSCITATION

1. Gradual Onset

2. Normal pupils

3. No focal neuro-
logic deficit
(or symmetrical
motor signs)
4. Asterixis
myoclonus,
tremor

1. Sudden Onset

2. Abnormal res-
piration often
at sunset.
3. Pupillary
abnormalities

4. "Crossed"
cranial nerve
palsies with
motor signs

1. Less Sudden Onset

2. Initial signs of
focal cerebral
dysfunction
3. Asymmetrical
motor signs

4. Progressive signs
of rostrocaudal
dysfunction

1. Active resistance
to lid opening
2. Eupnea or hyper-
ventilation

3. Normal pupils

4. Normal oculo-
vestibular
reflexes

METABOLIC
COMA

1. Toxicology
screen
2. Blood
Chemistry
a) Glucose
b) BUN,
serum
creatinine
c) LFT
d) Serum
electrolytes,
Ca + 2
e) Arterial
blood gases

INFRATENTORIAL
STRUCTURAL
LESION

CT

Operable
Lesion
(e.g. cerebellar
hemorrhage)

Neurosurgical
Care

Inoperable
Lesion
(e.g. pontine
hemorrhage)

Supportive
Care

SUPRATENTORIAL
STRUCTURAL
LESION

CT

Normal

LP

Meningitis
Antibiotics

Blood

SAH
Neurosurgical Consult

Normal
Supportive
Care

Operable
Lesion
(e.g.
subdural)

Neuro-
surgical
Care

PSYCHIATRIC
UNRESPONSIVENESS

Psychiatric Referral

Inoperable
Lesion
(e.g. cerebral
infarct)

Supportive
Care

"You see, even when all the evidence points to some other diagnosis, Jerry still checks the blood glucose level and pushes the thiamine, glucose, and Narcan®. That's the protocol. Period. He does this without fail in every case of coma and he does it within the first minute of the prehospital encounter," Frank explained.

"And if the patient doesn't improve with this therapy?" I asked.

"Then, the 60-Second EMT continues supportive measures with special attention to the airway and prevention of aspiration," explained Frank. "And, finally, if *any* neurologic impairment—confusion, combative behavior, amnesia, seizures, focal deficit, or obtundation—occurs in the setting of trauma, immediate transport and attention to the ABCs is of the utmost importance. When these signs are present, coma can be just around the corner. Focusing on these priorities is what separates the 60-Second EMT from the rest of the pack."

And it was Frank Zimmer's association with Jerry Donnelly—and his 60-Second Coma Exam—that separated *him* from the rest of the pack. With this program under his belt, he had clearly moved to the head of the class.

COMA

I. As always, vigorously attend to the ABCs: **A**irway control, ensurance of adequate **B**reathing and ventilation, and attendance to the **C**irculatory status of the patient.

Remember that the "C" also includes cervical spine control in a patient with coma of undetermined etiology: about 15% of all head-trauma patients will have coexisting significant cervical spinal injury. From a practical perspective, all head-trauma patients should be assumed to have coexisting C-spine injury until proven otherwise.

II. Remember the trio: thiamine, $D_{50}W$, and naloxone (also remember to save a sample of blood for a "pre-$D_{50}W$" glucose determination). A partial response to each may signify:

A. An extreme condition (e.g., extreme hypoglycemia or narcotic overdose).

B. More than one cause for the coma.

1. Chemical intoxication and coexistent head trauma.

2. Multiple drug ingestion (most overdoses fit into this category).

3. Other organ system involvement, such as shock, aspiration, or sepsis.

C. Overdose with a drug that requires higher dosage of naloxone to reverse—especially propoxyphene (Darvon®) or pentazocine (Talwin®).

III. Not all narcotic overdoses cause coma, respiratory depression, and pinpoint pupils.

A. Meperidine (Demerol®) overdose can result in dilated pupils and also can cause seizures. Propoxyphene (Darvon®) can cause the same reactions as meperidine.

B. If the patient has been hypoxic too long, fixed and dilated pupils can result from cerebral hypoxia.

IV. Remember the *"lucid interval"*: Those patients who "talked and died" will frequently have intracranial hematoma (either epidural or subdural). The fact that they "talked" before they lost consciousness implies that these patients have intact brain function and that the coma is secondary to the bleeding. These are patients for whom you can make a difference—by rapid evacuation to a facility with the capacity for immediate neurosurgical intervention.

V. *Never* assume that because a patient smells of alcohol, he or she is comatose from the alcohol alone. Alcoholics also have a much higher incidence of the following diseases, which also produce coma:

A. Head trauma.

B. Seizures: The coma may in actuality really be a postictal state.

C. Metabolic acidosis: in the most extreme cases, metabolic acidosis can cause coma and coexisting Kussmaul respirations (rapid, deep, and regular).

D. GI hemorrhage with shock and secondary coma.

E. Infections, including meningitis and sepsis (which can produce coma by secondary shock).

F. Hypoglycemia.

G. Encephalopathy.

H. Ingestion of toxic alcohol substitutes or other drugs.

VI. Be vigilant in *continuously* reevaluating your patients. Conditions can either improve from your interventions or they can dramatically worsen.

A. Do not cause an inordinate delay in transporting your patient.

B. Remember that naloxone can be injected either SL, IM, SC, or ET.

C. Glucagon, although not a substitute for glucose, is a hormone that directly antagonizes the actions of insulin. It can be given intramuscularly (average dose: 1 mg) and can occasionally save your patient's life or brain function (or both).

VII. **60-Second Triage:**

A. **ALS** backup should be called for any comatose patient.

B. **BLS** transport is permissible in a few circumstances:
  1. Rapid and total response to $D_{50}W$ in a known diabetic patient.
  2. Rapid and total response to naloxone in known narcotic overdose. Care should be taken if transport times are more than 20 minutes because naloxone will have passed its peak effect and the patient can then lapse into coma.
  3. Known isolated head trauma when transport time to the hospital is shorter than the time until arrival of the nearest ALS unit.

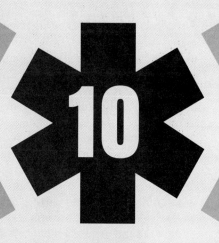

10

The 60-Second
Toxicology Exam

indy DeMent was one of the most respected EMTs in the state. She had been a licensed practical nurse for many years before becoming involved in prehospital care. Donnelly had told me that her special areas of interest were toxicology and psychiatry, two fields that EMTs know are frequently interrelated. Furthermore, she spent much of her off-duty time tending the hotline at the Regional Poison Control Center. I could not wait to meet her.

I introduced myself to the receptionist at Poison Control and told her that I had an appointment with Cindy.

"She's expecting you," was the answer. She ushered me into the communications room where Cindy was talking on the phone with an EMT who was caring for a poisoned patient in the field. I waited near the window and listened to the conversation.

"Let me make sure I have this straight," Cindy said in a professional tone of voice. "You're with a 5-year-old child who got into a Tylenol bottle and ingested between fifteen and twenty 325-mg acetaminophen tablets about 20 minutes ago?"

She seemed sharp as a tack.

"That's right," the EMT answered over the phone's loudspeaker, as Cindy jotted down some notes.

"What is the patient's level of consciousness?" she inquired.

Cindy glanced over at me to acknowledge my presence. She raised her right index finger to indicate that she would be with me in a moment.

"The kid looks alert and happy," answered the EMT. "He's running around the living room smashing his Barney doll against the wall."

"Sounds as if his mental status is just fine," she offered with a sense of humor. She then inquired wisely, "Are you sure the patient hasn't ingested any other toxins? We want to be certain the child hasn't ingested any strong acids, alkalis, hydrocarbons, or anything else that could depress his level of consciousness."

"No," the paramedic answered. "The mother seems very reliable and she's sure that the only thing that's been tampered with is the Tylenol® bottle."

"All right. Go ahead and give the child 15 cc of ipecac by mouth and a glass of water," Cindy relayed. "Be sure you have an emesis basin handy to catch any pill fragments, and bring what's left in the bottle to the emergency department."

Cindy hung up the phone, turned to another member of the staff, and said, "Mark, I'm going to be in conference for the next hour or so. Do you think you could manage the phones until I get back?"

"No problem," Mark answered, putting on a pair of earphones.

Cindy strolled over to where I was sitting, put out her hand and gave mine a firm shake. "Glad to meet you," she said. "Anyone who likes Jerry Donnelly is a friend of mine. I'll be glad to help you with your research in any way I can."

"Another member of the Jerry Donnelly Fan Club," I thought to myself. It seemed they were everywhere. And the more people I talked to, the more I felt I was on the trail of some EMT cult.

"How did you first run into Donnelly?" I asked Cindy.

"He's my cousin," Cindy responded with a grin.

That was the last thing I had expected to hear.

And then she added, "Actually, Jerry's my *third* cousin. But his 60-Second EMT Program has so much going for it, I like to claim him as part of the immediate family."

"Hmmm, I see," I said, not knowing what to say next. It was the only reply I could muster.

"Jerry and I developed an EMT rotation at the Regional Poison Control Center," Cindy continued, clarifying her professional ties with Donnelly. "It's been one of the most popular teaching modules in our EMT training program."

I sensed I was on the right track. I'd heard about Donnelly's success in developing a 60-Second Toxicology Exam, and my hunch was that much of the work had been done with Cindy DeMent. I could hardly wait for her to spell out the specifics of his approach.

"We have spent a lot of time teaching EMTs and paramedics the basic principles of assessing and managing individuals who have been exposed to hazardous materials and ingested poisons," Cindy explained. "In fact, for the past two years, Jerry and I have been going out in the field to train and supervise prehospital care providers in poison management right on the spot. It seems to be the most effective way of getting across the fundamentals of the 60-second approach."

"And what are the key elements of Donnelly's approach to the poisoned patient?" I asked.

"Let's take the Tylenol® ingestion I just handled over the phone," she began. "After getting some essential information about the case, I eventually recommended that the EMT administer ipecac. This can be a critical action in managing the poisoned patient; in fact, it's one of the few potentially lifesaving agents EMTs can administer to patients who have ingested a toxin. Also, with reliable history, some of these patients may not need to be taken to the hospital. But ipecac is not without its risks. For example, ipecac is effective within 30 minutes of toxin ingestion; use after 30 minutes is not recommended. It is very important that EMTs know what the indications and contraindications are. If not used properly, the complications can be horrendous."

Ipecac is effective within 30 minutes of toxin ingestion.

"Is there a 60-second formula to guide its use?" I wondered.

"Of course!" she replied. "Donnelly teaches his 60-Second EMTs several criteria for ipecac administration, all of which can be established within the first minute of patient contact."

I began to see the beauty of his 60-second system. Like Hamlet, the EMT is faced with a critical decision when treating every conscious patient with a toxic ingestion. "To administer ipecac or not to administer it, that is the question." Apparently Donnelly had devised a simple set of rules for resolving the issue.

"For example," Cindy went on, "ipecac should *not* be given to patients who are unconscious or who are suspected of taking medications that might lead to a rapidly diminishing level of consciousness." And then she explained, "A thorough history of the ingestion is crucial for making this decision. Similarly, ipecac should never be given to patients who are having seizures or who have a poor gag reflex. Ipecac should not be used in the field to induce vomiting in patients who have ingested acids, alkalis (lye), silver nitrate, iodides, strychnine, or petroleum products. Finally, we ask that our EMTs contact the poison control center whenever possible before administering ipecac."

"It's really a very simple way to approach critical action," I commented.

"That's right, it is," she agreed. "And once the EMT has admin-

---

Contraindications for Ipecac Use

Do not administer ipecac to patients who are:
  Unconscious
  Seizing
  Without gag reflex
  Suspected of having ingested acids, alkali, silver nitrate, iodides, strychnine or petroleum products

istered ipecac—30 ml for adults and 15 ml for children over one year of age—we recommend that oral fluids and ambulation be used to enhance the emetic action. We also emphasize that the gag reflex may not always be a reliable indicator of whether the patient can protect his or her airway. EMTs should always stand by with suction and have the patient sitting or in the recovery position after ipecac is given."

"Cindy, what about the ipecac vs. activated charcoal/sorbitol controversy?" I asked. "There is a growing dispute as to which agent should be used in the field. Usually, ipecac is the treatment of choice for 'home care.' If hospital transport is needed, activated charcoal/sorbitol at 1 to 2 g/kg is preferred. If the ingestion is recent and the history reliable, we still may order ipecac for patients being transported."

Donnelly's 60-second approach to prehospital ipecac administration was really sound. And practical. I could see why he was so famous for his system. But there was a hitch. In practice, many overdoses produce patients who already have a depressed level of consciousness when the EMT arrives at the scene. Ipecac or charcoal administration is out of the question in such cases.

"What about patients who exhibit depressed levels of consciousness and can't take ipecac or charcoal for that reason?" I asked. "And what about patients who have ingested an unknown toxin, or toxins, and there is no one around to give a history?" It seemed to me that the 60-Second EMT would have to be able to handle these situations as well.

> EMTs should always stand by with suction and have the patient sitting or in the recovery position after ipecac is given.

"The 60-second approach is very different for those patients, but it's just as effective," Cindy was quick to point out. "Let me tell you about a case that may help answer your question. Jerry and I were called to see an unresponsive young man in the Bowery. We pulled the rig up to one of those seedy flophouses, you know the kind of place where vices outnumber virtues by ten to one. In a small, dingy room lit by a single light bulb, we found a 25-year-old male lying on the floor. He was cyanotic, had shallow respirations, and was unresponsive."

"How did the 60-second approach apply in his case?" I asked with a spark of curiosity.

"Well, it ought to be clear from the outset that with patients who have depressed level of consciousness, the 60-second ipecac/

activated charcoal pathway is not the place to start," she explained. "In some cases like this, Donnelly uses the 60-second approach for the *unconscious* toxic patient. It's very different.

"When I finish telling you about this case, I think you'll get the point," Cindy continued. "I immediately took steps to control the patient's airway. At the same time, I saw Jerry's eyes scanning the patient's body and darting across the room at lightning speed. He discovered that the patient had pinpoint pupils. Then he smelled the patient's breath and detected alcohol. He felt to see if the patient's skin was dry or clammy and looked for signs of urinary and fecal incontinence.

" 'He's got track marks on his arms, there are syringes in the sink, and there's an empty bottle of vodka on the window sill.' Jerry spoke with computer-like precision within 20 seconds of entering the room. 'He's unresponsive, so let's give him two amps of Narcan (naloxone, 2 mg), 100 mg of thiamine, and 50 ml of 50% dextrose.' He must have ordered these within 10 seconds. I couldn't believe how fast things were happening."

"That gives him another 30 seconds, and his minute will be up," I added with a chuckle. "So what happened then?" I asked.

"The patient's respirations improved dramatically," Cindy reported. "At that point, he was awake enough to tell us he'd shot some heroin and that he'd been drinking. And that's all he told us. With his sensorium apparently improving, I was satisfied that the Narcan had done its job. But his level of consciousness was still somewhat depressed—from the alcohol, I assumed—so we put him on a cardiac monitor as a precaution. It showed a sinus tachycardia with wide QRS complexes and frequent PVCs. Jerry looked at the monitor somewhat puzzled. I wasn't sure why. Then, within 30 seconds or so after loading the patient onto the stretcher, the patient became apneic and unresponsive again.

" 'There's something strange going on here,' Jerry said as he administered more Narcan. Again, the patient improved dramatically. I admired Jerry's quick thinking in this situation."

"So you transported the patient at that point?" I asked.

"Not quite," she said with a twinkle in her eye. "In all overdoses, the 60-second approach encourages the EMT to make a vigorous search for evidence that other toxins might be involved. This means looking for pill bottles, prescriptions, pill fragments, and drug paraphernalia. It also means extracting as much information as you can from bystanders—remembering, of course, that their information may not always be reliable."

"But in this case, everything pointed to the heroin and alcohol overdose," I offered. "There was really nothing else you could do."

"Initially it seemed that way, but when the guy went out a second time, the plot began to thicken." Cindy said. "Donnelly always stresses that the EMT has to assume that all overdoses are *polypharmacy* overdoses—that is, they are caused by more than one agent—until proven otherwise. That's part of his 60-second approach."

> Assume that all overdoses are *polypharmacy* overdoses—that is, they are caused by more than one agent— until proven otherwise.

"How did that affect what you did next?" I wanted to know.

"Well, after checking to ensure that the patient was stabilized enough to delay transport, Jerry quickly scoured the room. He looked through the drug cabinet, drawers, and closets—in every nook and cranny he could think of—and just when I thought that we'd gotten everything we were going to get in this case, Jerry lifted up a grungy mattress and discovered two empty pill bottles. One was for Darvon and the other was for tricyclic antidepressants—Elavil, I think. I couldn't believe it."

"I bet finding those bottles really changed the complexion of the case," I marveled.

"That's for sure. Once we knew that we were probably dealing with a Darvon (propoxyphene) ingestion, Jerry gave him six more amps of Narcan to make sure we had sufficient narcotic antagonism. As you know, propoxyphene can require large doses of naloxone for reversal. Finding the bottle of tricyclic antidepressants helped explain the patient's PVCs and, also, why his mental status remained compromised after the Narcan. We hyperventilated the patient's lungs and gave him some IV fluids and 75 mEq of NaHCO$_3$. As Jerry gave the bicarb, I saw the QRS complexes narrow and PVCs subside. The patient's LOC increased, and he was conscious and alert upon arrival at the ED.

"After the call, I asked Jerry why bicarb was indicated. He explained that by creating alkalosis, you reduce the cardiac toxicity of tricyclic anti-depressants."

This was an extraordinary example of Donnelly's 60-second approach at work. His every move was executed like clockwork and each unexpected twist in the case was eventually explained—sometimes, even resolved—by a critical action that was part of the 60-Second Assessment of Toxicology. I tried to summarize what I had just learned.

"As I understand it, then," I said to Cindy, "Donnelly's 60-second approach to the unconscious patient with a toxic ingestion is to manage the ABCs—especially the airway—start an IV line, and administer thiamine, D_{50}, and Narcan. After the primary and secondary survey, it's time to make a rapid, thorough search of the patient and his environment, looking for clues to suggest *all* the possible toxins that might have played a role in the patient's condition. When bystanders are available, they should be pumped for information."

"You've got it," she said enthusiastically. "And remember, you can frequently get some idea of what the ingested drug is from the patient's physical signs and symptoms. I think Jerry's 60-second method is very helpful in making this distinction. He lumps drug ingestion into the 'uppers' and the 'downers.' The uppers—stimulants such as cocaine, amphetamines, tricyclic antidepressants, and anticholinergics—tend to cause pupillary dilation (mydriasis), tachycardia, hypertension, arrhythmias, hyperkinetic behavioral changes, and seizures. They can cause respiratory distress. The downers—a large class of drugs including sleeping pills, phenobarbital, diazepam (Valium®), and cholinergics—generally cause profound mental depression and respiratory compromise. Although supportive management, especially control of the airway, is the mainstay of prehospital care for both groups, it's frequently helpful to know which class of drugs you're dealing with."

> **Control of the airway is the mainstay of prehospital care for drug overdoses.**

"The Uppers"	"The Downers"
Cocaine	Sleeping pills
Amphetamines	Phenobarbital
Tricyclic antidepressants	Valium
Anticholinergics	Cholinergics
may cause	**can cause**
Pupilary dilation	Profound mental depression
Tachycardia	Respiratory compromise
Hypertension	
Arrhythmias	
Hyperkinetic behavioral changes	
Seizures	
Respiratory distress	

Specific Antidotes for Drug Overdose

POISON	ANTIDOTE
Acetaminophen	N-acetylcysteine (Mucomyst)
Anticholinergic agents	Physostigmine (Antilirium)
Carbon monoxide	100% oxygen
Cyanide	Sodium nitrate, sodium thiosulfate
Ferrous salts	Deferoxamine
Lead	EDTA*
Mercury (arsenic gold)	BAL*
Methanol (ethylene glycol)	Ethanol
Narcotics	Naloxone (Narcan)
Nitrites	Methylene blue
Organophosphates	Atropine, pralidoxime

*EDTA = calcium disodium edetate; BAL = British anti-Lewisite.

Donnelly's 60-second system offered a sound approach to the use of supportive measures and naloxone in the management of poisonings. I knew, however, that there were other antidotes in use and wondered whether the 60-Second EMT had included these in his scheme. Cindy answered just before I could ask my question.

"But that's still not the whole story. There are situations—actually, they're the exceptions rather than the rule—that call for very specific antidotes in the prehospital setting. While it is true that most ingestions and poisonings do not have specific antidotes, there are a few that do, and Jerry includes them in his 60-second approach to poison management. Sometimes these specific antidotes can be lifesaving, so it's critical that the 60-Second EMT be familiar with their rational use. I'm referring to agents like calcium chloride and glucagon."

"Hey, wait a minute! Calcium chloride is not used anymore."

Cindy answered, "Calcium chloride, although no longer used in cardiac arrest, is the antidote for calcium channel blocker overdose."

"I get it. Now that lots of people are taking these meds for hypertension, arrhythmias, and headaches, an antidote for these drugs is necessary."

Cindy smiled and said, "Let me give you an example. Jerry told me about a case where a 65-year-old male was found by his family to be unresponsive.

> Calcium chloride, although no longer used in cardiac arrest, is the antidote for calcium channel blocker overdose.

Upon Jerry's arrival, the patient was unconscious—responsive only to deep pain. His pulse was 55, respirations 8, and BP 78/40.

"BVM ventilation with 100% O_2 was started, blood drawn, and IV access obtained. Jerry immediately instituted the thiamine/D_{50}/Narcan protocol with no results. As ET intubation was performed, Jerry noticed an empty bottle of Calan SR. He quickly realized that we were dealing with a possible calcium channel blocker–overdose. Worse than that, since this involved "SR" (slow-release) capsules, this OD might have happened hours before.

"So what did Jerry do? He quickly ran IV fluids wide open and gave 1 gm of calcium chloride IV. The patient's BP increased to 100/60 and the pulse increased to 80. During transport, the patient started responding to verbal command. Once again, Jerry used his 60-Second EMT Program to handle a critical and confusing case."

Profile of Fatality Rates Among Elderly Patients with Toxic Ingestion

	NUMBER OF GERIATRIC FATALITIES (%)
Analgesics	40 (19.4)
Cardiovascular drugs	32 (16.5)
Antidepressants	27 (13.9)
Asthma therapies	19 (9.8)
Cleaning substances	14 (7.2)
Gases and fumes	12 (6.2)
Alcohols/glycols	9 (4.6)
Sedative-hypnotics	9 (4.6)
Chemicals (cyanide, acid)	8 (4.1)
Insecticides/pesticides	4 (2.1)
Antipsychotics	3 (1.6)
Hydrocarbon solvents	3 (1.6)
Heavy metals (arsenic)	2 (1.0)
Miscellaneous	12 (6.2)

Specific Drugs Causing Overdose in the Elderly

Theophylline	Amitriptyline
Aspirin	Alkaline cleaners
Digoxin	Ethylene glycol
Acetaminophen	Imipramine
Carbon monoxide	Verapamil

TOXICOLOGY

I. Conscious vs. Unconscious:
   In treating the obtunded or comatose patient:
   A. Manage the ABCs.
   B. Administer thiamine, $D_{50}W$, and naloxone with few, if any, exceptions.
   C. Always consider the possibility of multiple drug ingestion.
   D. Consider the administration of at least 2 mg of naloxone, and even more in the event of only a partial patient response of the patient (especially with the possibility of Darvon [propoxyphene] or Talwin® [pentazocine] overdose).
   E. Never forget the possibility of concurrent head injury.

II. Ipecac is the primary agent for home care. Most patients needing hospital transport should be treated with activated charcoal/sorbitol (1 to 2 g/kg PO)

III. Ipecac should not be given to the following patients:
   A. Unconscious patients or those with ingestion of substances potentially causing rapid deterioration of consciousness (e.g., tricyclic antidepressants, propranolol).
   B. Patients with no gag reflex.
   C. Patients who have ingested acid and alkalis.
   D. Those who have ingested hydrocarbons (petroleum products), strychnine, iodides, or silver nitrate.

IV. Always search the premises for pill bottles, prescriptions, pill fragments, and drug paraphernalia. Bring these in for any unknown drug ingestion or suicide attempt (regardless of what the patient who attempted may tell you).

V. The "Uppers":
   A. Include: cocaine, amphetamines, phencyclidine (PCP), tricyclic antidepressants, and anticholinergics.

C. Overdoses of calcium channel blockers (Calan®, Procardia®) and beta blockers (Lopressor®, Tenormin®) are more prevalent.

   1. Calcium chloride is the antidote for calcium channel blocker–overdose. Aggressive fluid therapy and dopamine may also be necessary. Atropine can be used for bradycardia but its results vary.

   2. Beta-agonist agents and glucagon are beneficial in symptomatic beta-blocker overdose. Higher doses may be needed to counteract the substance.

VIII. **60-Second Triage:**

A. **BLS** transport can be accomplished if the patient has ingested a known drug or toxin of low poison potential (after appropriate consultation with the base station physician or the poison center) and has:

   1. Normal vital signs.

   2. Clear and normal mental status.

B. **ALS** transport is essential for patients with any of the following:

   1. Abnormal mental status (ranging from coma to delirium to seizures).

   2. Abnormal vital signs.

   3. Any of the conditions in I that contraindicate the use of ipecac or activated charcoal/sorbitol.

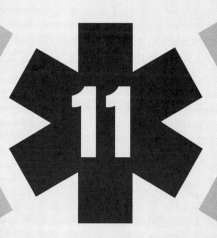

The 60-Second
Special Lecture:
Hazardous Materials

Bob Livingston, my supervisor at the station, had heard that I was researching the 60-Second EMT during my time off. He tapped me on the shoulder one afternoon as I was cleaning the rig after a long shift.

"I hear you're interested in learning all you can about Jerry Donnelly," he grinned. "I thought you might be interested in this." He held out a red binder. "I attended an excellent continuing education workshop on Hazardous Materials. . . ."

"Let me guess," I interrupted. "It was led by the 60-Second EMT himself!"

"None other," Bob nodded. "Maybe my notes can give you some insights to the man."

"Thanks, boss. I really appreciate this."

Bob was right. The information was excellent. In fact, I stayed up late reading despite the fact that I had just worked a 12-hour shift.

INTRODUCTION

Hazardous materials and toxic chemical exposure are byproducts of a technologic and industrial society. The Environmental Protection Agency has listed more than 50,000 products as harmful or potentially harmful on exposure. Exposure can occur anywhere in the manufacturing process, transportation, storage, or application of these products.

ROLE OF HAZMAT

Large-scale exposure incidents, such as toxic spills on freeways, train derailments, manufacturing explosions, or fires, include prehospital care providers as a part of an integrated team. Another crucial component of this team is an organization of hazardous materials–response units known as HAZMAT or HAZMAT units. The role of HAZMAT includes obtaining information about hazardous material used at a given site, scheduling inspections to determine safety hazards, and developing a resource inventory for technical assistance, supplies, and equipment.

At a scene of hazardous materials exposure, equipment should be available for detection of hazardous materials and personal protection. There should also be containment materials, such as plugs, sealants, fire retardants, and absorbing agents. Resuscitation equipment and antidotes for specific exposure should be available for treatment. Initial rescue and clearing of victims from the scene will often require protective gear and self-contained breathing apparatus.

AT THE SCENE

Paramedics arriving at a scene should give priority to protecting themselves. This includes identifying potential hazardous materials incidents.

Paramedics arriving at a scene should give priority to protecting themselves.

Buildings have codes or placards (see below), and the Department of Transportation has shipping labels that indicate health risk, fire risk, or reactivity of products in use. MSDS sheets are available and should be obtained for transportation incidents. The presence of odors, fumes, gas leaks, or spills, or identification of hazardous materials placards or shipping papers are clues that should lead to recognition of hazardous materials and coordination with a poison control center and/or the hazardous materials team.

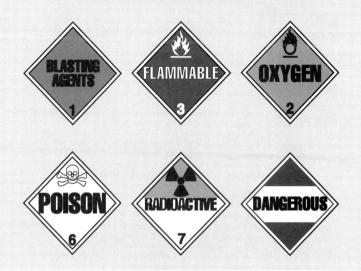

POISONS	ANTIDOTES
Acetaminophen	N-acetylcysteine (NAC, Mucomyst)
Anticholinergics	Physostigmine
Arsenic	Dimercaprol (BAL), D-penicillamine
Beta-adrenergic antagonists	Glucagon
Benzodiazepine	Flumazenil
Botulism	Botulinum antitoxin (ABE trivalent)
Cadmium	$CaNa_2$ EDTA, D-penicillamine
Calcium channel blocker	Calcium chloride
Cardiac glycosides	Digoxin immune FAB (Digibind)
Carbamates	Atropine, pralidoxime (2-PAM)
Chlorine gas	Sodium bicarbonate
Cobalt	$CaNa_2$ EDTA
Copper	Dimercaprol (BAL), D-penicillamine, $CaNa_2$ EDTA
Coumarin derivatives	Vitamin K_1 (Phytonadione)
Cyanide	Amyl nitrite, sodium nitrate, sodium thiosulfate, oxygen, hydroxocobalamin
Tricyclic antidepressants	Sodium bicarbonate
Ethylene glycol	Ethanol, pyridoxine, thiamine
Hydrazines	Pyridoxine (Vitamin B_6)
Hydrogen sulfide	Amyl nitrite, sodium nitrite, oxygen
Hydrofluoric acid	Calcium gluconate, magnesium sulfate

EXPOSURE

The EMT should consider four basic patterns and be aware of his/her own exposure risk. These patterns are (1) dermal exposure resulting in local effects, (2) dermal exposure resulting in systemic effects, (3) inhalation resulting in local effects, and (4) inhalation resulting in systemic effects.

The EMT should be aware of his/her own exposure risk.

DERMAL EXPOSURE/LOCAL EFFECT

Dermal exposure with local effect results primarily from acids and alkalis, but about 25,000 different products are estimated to cause chemical burns. The appearance of such burns is similar

POISONS	ANTIDOTES
Hypoglycemics	Dextrose, glucagon, hydrocortisone, diazoxide
Iron	Deferoxamine
Inorganic mercury	Dimercaprol (BAL), dimercaptosuccinic acid (DMSA), D-penicillamine
Lead	Dimercaprol (BAL), CaNa$_2$ EDTA, dimercaptosuccinic acid (DMSA), D-penicillamine
Magnesium	Calcium gluconate
Methanol	Ethanol, folinic acid (Leucovorin)
Methemoglobinemia	Methylene blue
Methotrexate	Folinic acid (Leucovorin)
Mushrooms	
Clitocybe/inocybe	Atropine
Amanita phalloides	Penicillin G, silibinin, silimaryn
Gyromitra esculenta	Pyridoxine
Neuroleptics (extrapyramidal symptoms)	Diphenhydramine Benztropine
Phenothiazines	
Butyrophenones	
Thioxanthenes	
Metoclopramide	
Opioids	Naloxone
Zinc	CaNa$_2$ EDTA, dimercaprol (BAL)

to that of thermal burns, but the injury is caused by chemical reactivity with tissue, rather than by heat. One consequence is that chemical injuries, which initially appear to be mild, can progress over time to extensive tissue damage—much more so than can thermal injuries, which do not worsen once they are removed from the heat source.

Field management begins with eliminating the exposing agent.

Field management begins with eliminating the exposing agent. Clothing that contains chemicals should be removed. Any solid material should be wiped off or debrided. This is important, especially for products such as metallic sodium, potassium, and phosphorus. Lavage should follow for 15 minutes if the patient is not otherwise injured and in need of immediate transport.

CASE REPORT

A glass etcher at work was splashed with hydrofluoric acid over his arm and hand. He washed out the affected areas but still had pain. Paramedics were contacted for transport. The MSDS sheet was obtained, Poison Control Center was contacted, and a gel was made with calcium gluconate and Lubriderm® and placed over the victim's hand and arm before transport. This significantly reduced later tissue damage.

DERMAL EXPOSURE/SYSTEMIC EFFECT

Most pesticides have a high rate of absorption, even through intact skin.

Dermal exposure with systemic toxicity is less common than local injury because intact skin provides a barrier to most compounds. Concomitant skin damage from fire or open wounds can greatly increase toxicity of normally nonabsorbed materials. Most pesticides have a high rate of absorption, even through intact skin. This absorption can also occur on exposed hands that are used to examine patients or remove clothing.

Pentachlorophenol is a potentially harmful agricultural product that is widely used to prevent fungal and insect damage to wood products and other organic materials.

Pentachlorophenol, when it is absorbed, breaks the link between energy production of body cells, and use by tissue. With such injury to the system, metabolism continues but no useful cellular work takes place. Significant exposure leads to high fever, agitation, and cardiac dysfunction.

Treatment consists of eliminating the source, removing all contaminated clothing, copious irrigation, careful cardiac monitoring, and transport.

INHALATION TOXICITY/LOCAL EFFECT

Inhalation of toxic chemicals with local toxicity refers to damage of the airway or mucous membrane, leading to respiratory distress or hypoxia. The number of products causing inhalation/systemic toxicity is much greater than that of any other category of toxic exposure. Chemical spills, fires, poorly ventilated enclosed areas, and traffic tollbooths are just a few examples of situations in which inhalation toxicity can occur.

Initial management includes supplemental oxygen, cardiac monitoring, and placement of IV. Irritation of the nose or mouth, watering or burning of the eyes (which suggests mucosal injury), hoarseness, barking cough, severe facial burns, or nasal burns are all clues to potential upper-airway tissue damage. Agitation, tachypnea, stridor, or wheezes upon auscultation are clues to lower-airway injury. Injured patients need careful observation for possible airway closure and the need for intubation.

Chemicals such as chlorine and sulfate compounds cause upper- and lower-airway difficulties.

Chemicals such as chlorine and sulfate compounds cause upper- and lower-airway difficulties. In contact with tissue water, these chemicals convert to their component acids, hydrochloric and sulfuric acids, respectively. The upper airway may tolerate this exposure, but significant alveolar injury is certain, with pulmonary edema and bronchospasm. Fume exposure causing watery or burning eyes and paroxysmal coughing, chest burning or tightness, rales, wheezes, or rhonchi (see Chap. 12: 60-Second Respiratory Exam) suggests lower-airway injury. Patients should be removed from the scene and their eyes irrigated if patient-stability allows. High-flow oxygen should be given and IV should be placed and kept open. To prevent overhydration and worsening of pulmonary edema, fluid challenge should be avoided unless needed for other reasons.

INHALATION TOXICITY/SYSTEMIC EFFECT

Central nervous system and cardiac toxicity occur from hypoxic injury and specific toxic events. Confusion and agitation may progress to coma and seizures. Management should follow protocol. Cardiac toxicity should be treated according to protocol except in cases of exposure to fluoronated hydrocarbons such as trichloroethylene or carbon tetrachloride. These are directly irritating to the heart and are arrythmogenic. **Administration of epinephrine or sympathomimetics for bronchospasm potentiates this effect and can lead to cardiac arrest.**

A major presenting symptom of victims at a fire scene is inadequate oxygen in the lungs and blood, or hypoxia. Differing immediate causes for hypoxia provide different rationales for particular treatments:

(1) Reduction of ambient O_2 as a result of oxygen consumption by

fire: Remove victim from the environment and apply
supplemental oxygen;

(2) Mechanical displacement of oxygen in the lungs by carbon
dioxide or other combustion products: Remove victim and
apply supplemental oxygen;

(3) Upper-airway injury, thermal or caustic: Remove victim from
the scene, apply supplemental oxygen—humidified if
possible—and consider early intubation;

(4) Lower-airway injury—bronchospasm or pulmonary edema. Apply
supplemental oxygen by bag-valve-mask respiration or PEEP
with intubation;

(5) Reduced oxygen-carrying by blood or reduced oxygen uptake by
tissue, primarily with carboxyhemoglobin or cyanide: Apply
oxygen and consider specific antidotes for cyanide toxicity.

Carbon monoxide is present at all fires and has no odor or
taste. All fire victims should receive supplemental oxygen with
100% O_2 especially if they are in an enclosed area. Persisting
confusion, obtundation, or coma without
evidence of a traumatic cause should lead to
transfer of the patient to a facility with a
hyperbaric chamber, if possible. A high oxygen
saturation does not rule out carbon
monoxide toxicity.

Confusion, stupor, coma, and cardiopulmonary arrest occur rapidly in significant cyanide exposure.

Hydrogen cyanide is a product of nitrogen-
containing organic polymers, which are
formed in the construction of such products
as furniture and carpets. Confusion, stupor, coma, and
cardiopulmonary arrest occur rapidly in significant cyanide
exposure. The presence of cyanide can be determined by HAZMAT
units. Cyanide is always suspected when materials burn. Red
venous blood appears in a person with cyanide toxicity because
the tissue exchange of oxygen is blocked and oxygenated blood
carries into the venous circulation. Amyl nitrate and sodium
nitrite (provided in the cyanide kit) convert hemoglobin to
methemoglobin. Cyanide releases from tissues and binds to this.
The administration of thiosulfate to a victim binds the cyanide
from hemoglobin and converts it to thiocyanate, which is less
toxic and is readily excreted.

Field administration of the cyanide kit is appropriate with base
station— or poison control—contact for isolated cyanide toxicity
or spills.

CONCLUSION

Supportive therapy, self-protection, use of specific antidotes when available, and obtaining MSDS sheets or product labels when possible are the ground rules in hazardous materials exposure–incidents.

(1) Protect yourself.

(2) Coordinate with HAZMAT or PCC.

(3) Recognize toxicologic patterns:

(a) Dermal exposure with local toxicity: acids and alkalis.

(b) Dermal exposure with systemic toxicity: pesticides, pentachlorophenol.

(c) Inhalation exposure with local toxicity: hot air, chlorine.

(d) Inhalation exposure with systemic toxicity: carbon tetrachloride, cyanide, carbon monoxide.

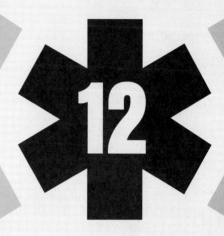

The 60-Second
Respiratory Exam

eople in the EMS community described Mark Christenson as zany and brilliant. Before Christenson became a paramedic, he had a reputation as quite a car enthusiast. He was especially "into" vintage cars, such as '57 Thunderbird two-seaters in perfect condition. Or so Donnelly had told me on the phone the night before my meeting with Mark.

Christenson's own pride and joy was a 1956 Chevy—a museum piece painted aqua and fire-engine red and refurbished with white calf upholstery. As legend has it, every Sunday Mark would drive into remote rural areas looking for junked cars to restore. He would come back from these jaunts with Edsels, Studebakers, and Chevys in tow. Mostly, they were nothing but scrapheaps on their way to "car heaven"! Somehow, though, he would resuscitate these vehicles from top to bottom and turn them into dream machines. Breathe life into them, if you will.

Mark's magic with cars was known. Some of his cars had even made it into a traveling Smithsonian exhibit on the history of the American automobile. One day, about five years ago, he gave it all up. Just like that. Rumor had it that a close friend of his was killed driving that '56 Chevy. Mark changed, and within a month he was training to become a paramedic. He got together with Jerry Donnelly about three years ago, and since that time Christenson has tackled one of the most difficult areas of prehospital care: diagnosing and assessing respiratory emergencies. In that specialty his brilliance has shown.

The day I pulled up to his ramshackle bungalow, Mark was putting a final spit polish on his '59 Corvette. "I see this car stuff is still in your blood," I offered by way of introduction.

"Yeah, guess so." he said shyly. "But I've moved on to other things. I'm sure Donnelly has told you as much."

In fact, Donnelly had told me much more. He made it clear that Christenson was the man to see if I wanted to learn more about the 60-Second Approach to Respiratory Emergencies.

"Mark, the word is that with your help, Donnelly has developed a very precise approach to prehospital care of patients with shortness of breath. What specific issues does the 60-second approach address?" I asked.

"Well, for starters," he replied, "Donnelly, and most paramedics, for that matter, know how difficult it is to distinguish among different causes of respiratory distress. That's what convinced him to develop a 60-second plan for this common and, I might add, very anxiety-producing problem."

"What's the crux of rapid respiratory assessment as Donnelly sees it?" I inquired.

"I'm glad you asked, because there seems to be one central issue, and it comes up over and over again. In nontraumatic medical emergencies," explained Mark, "EMTs are often faced with the problem of distinguishing between cardiac and pulmonary causes of respiratory distress. Each of these disorders requires a different form of therapy, so it's critical for the EMT to know which entity he or she is dealing with."

> EMTs are often faced with the problem of distinguishing between cardiac and pulmonary causes of respiratory distress.

Christenson had hit the nail on the head. Every EMT I know has complained, at some point in their career, about the difficulty of distinguishing between congestive heart failure (CHF) and chronic obstructive pulmonary disease (COPD). It is a classic dilemma that paramedics find challenging on the one hand but, on the other, very stressful in the prehospital setting. In patients with respiratory distress, EMTs trained in advanced life support are faced with a difficult therapeutic decision. Do you give nitroglycerin, furosemide (Lasix®), and morphine to the patient with presumed cardiac-induced pulmonary edema? Or do you administer an inhaled bronchodilator to a patient thought to have worsening COPD or asthma? From an assessment point of view, untangling the subtleties of each condition presents a host of problems, so I asked Mark what Donnelly had to offer in this regard. His response, simple and clear, was a real eye opener.

> The 60-Second Respiratory Exam always stresses the importance of, first, an accurate history and, second, a rapid primary survey.

"In the 60-Second Respiratory Exam, Donnelly always stresses the importance of, first, an accurate history and, second, a rapid primary survey. You want to know very early in your contact with these patients, especially in elderly individuals who may already have established a pattern of complications caused by their underlying disease, whether or not there is a past history of congestive heart failure (CHF) or COPD. For example, Donnelly immediately asks if there have been previous episodes of congestive heart failure. This may seem obvious, but it's important. For example, if patients say 'Yes,' Donnelly then asks them if the symptoms they're having are similar to those experienced in past episodes. A patient may say something like 'Yeah, it feels like my lungs are filling up with fluid again.' This gives the 60-Second EMT a feel for the patient before going on to the physical exam."

"And what about patients with COPD?" I asked.

"The same principle applies," Mark said, taking a piece of lamb's wool from the glove compartment. "In patients with COPD, you want to know whether their attack of respiratory distress is similar to previous episodes in which their COPD worsened. For example, have environmental factors or an underlying viral illness made their COPD worse in recent days? Again, let the patient—and the history—be your first guide. That's central to the whole 60-second concept. Most patients give you histories that are helpful. In general, though not always, those with heart disease have respiratory distress caused by congestive heart failure. Those with COPD deteriorate from bronchoconstriction or poor airflow. 'When you hear hoofbeats,' as the old saying goes, 'think of horses first, not zebras.' "

I wondered whether the 60-second approach included any specific clues that the EMT could use once the patient's previous history had been established.

"Once you know the patient's past history, are there any other historical features that the 60-Second Respiratory Exam emphasizes?" I inquired.

"Absolutely," Christenson confirmed. "Within the first minute of contact you have to ask about compliance with medications. If cardiac patients tell you they haven't taken medications, or that they've run out of their diuretic (water pill), high blood pressure–medications, or heart pills (digoxin), there's a good chance their respiratory distress is caused by fluid overload and congestive heart failure."

"Are there possible medication changes for COPD patients that the 60-Second EMT should ask about?"

"Yes, there are, and of course you should ask them within the Golden Minute. For example, if the patient with COPD has stopped taking his bronchodilator, failed to refill his inhaler, or his steroid medications (used to treat severe cases of COPD) have recently been tapered off, the EMT has good reason to suspect that the COPD is worsening and can treat the patient accordingly. These are data the EMT can obtain early in the patient encounter.

Within 60 seconds, you can get a patient's medication history and decide if it points in a certain direction. Usually it does. Meanwhile, of course, you're stabilizing the patient with oxygen, sitting him upright, and reassuring him. These basic therapeutic measures are taken regardless of the underlying cause of respiratory distress."

> Stabilize the patient with oxygen, sit him upright, and reassure him.

"What about the physical exam?" I asked. "Isn't it often difficult to distinguish between cardiac and pulmonary causes of respiratory distress?"

"Yes, it is," he admitted.

"And isn't the picture frequently one of combined pulmonary *and* cardiac failure?"

"Yes."

"So what does the EMT do?"

"You've hit on something that Donnelly deals with in the 60-Second EMT Program," Christenson explained, as he gave the chrome detailing on his door an extra shine. "In fact, that's why Donnelly emphasizes certain features of the physical exam."

"What parts of the exam, in particular?"

"Well, patients with COPD can fall into one of two categories," Mark explained. "The emphysematous patients are called 'pink puffers,' and those with the bronchitic form of COPD are known as 'blue bloaters.' Both tend to have barrel chests. Pink puffers may have pursed lips, and sometimes their chest walls barely move. When you auscultate a patient with emphysema, you hear markedly diminished breath sounds. In severe cases, you may not be able to hear any breath sounds at all. In bronchitic patients, the EMT usually hears rhonchi and diffuse wheezes. And remember, patients with COPD can deteriorate suddenly. If they do, you have to listen again and be sure they still have *bilateral* breath sounds. If they lose breath sounds on one side, you have to suspect a pneumothorax. Patients with emphysema can rupture a bleb and col-

---

Patients with COPD

Emphysematous	Bronchitic
("Pink Puffers")	("Blue Bloaters")
Barrel chest	Barrel chest
Pursed lips	Rhonchi heard on auscultation
Little chest wall movement	Diffuse wheezes
Diminished breath sounds	

Patients with CHF	
Dyspneic	Jugular venous distension
Orthopneic	Peripheral edema
Tachypneic	Chest discomfort
Pink-tinged sputum (indicates	Cardiac arrhythmia
pulmonary edema)	Inspiratory rales or crackles

lapse a lung, so you've got to be on the lookout for a pneumothorax."

"How does the cardiac patient with CHF differ?" I pressed Christenson.

"Patients with CHF are, of course, also short of breath," Christenson said. "They are dyspneic, orthopneic (having worse trouble breathing when lying down than sitting up), and tachypneic, just like patients with chronic lung disease . But there are other clues. They may produce a pink-tinged sputum, which is characteristic of pulmonary edema. And they may have jugular venous distension, peripheral edema, and chest discomfort. They may have a cardiac arrhythmia. If they do, chances are excellent that you're dealing with congestive heart failure. Experienced paramedics can also detect inspiratory rales or crackles at the lung bases, a very good clue that CHF is the culprit. Appropriate therapy for CHF in these cases includes high-flow oxygen, sublingual or IV nitroglycerin, intravenous Lasix, and, perhaps, morphine sulfate."

From what I could gather, the 60-Second Respiratory Exam provided an excellent strategy for lumping patients into cardiac and pulmonary categories on the basis of a quick initial history and primary survey. That in itself was impressive, but I was curious as to how Donnelly applied the 60-second approach to patients with a history of *both* CHF and COPD. These are the patients that drive EMTs up the wall and create anxiety.

Appropriate therapy for CHF includes high-flow oxygen, sublingual or IV nitroglycerin, intravenous Lasix, and, perhaps, morphine sulfate.

So I put the question to Mark in very direct terms. "How does the 60-Second Respiratory Exam help the EMT isolate the underlying cause in patients with more complicated conditions—for example, those with both cardiac and pulmonary problems?"

"You've put your finger on the great challenge," Christenson confirmed. "And you've got to realize from the outset that even experienced physicians may struggle with diagnoses for this group. But maybe I can answer with a real-life example I saw Donnelly handle a few months back."

"Sure, go ahead," I said.

"We were called to see a 70-year-old man in respiratory distress," he began. "On arrival, we found that the patient had a respiratory rate of 30, was cyanotic, and was sitting bolt upright. His blood pressure was 184/110, his heart rate was 126, and he could barely complete a sentence with more than three words. Donnelly asked him if he had a previous history of COPD, and the patient said, 'Yeah, real bad . . . I've been using my inhaler.' "

"Did Donnelly give him some aerosolized bronchodilator?"

"Not yet," cautioned Christenson. "Jerry wanted a little more history. Meanwhile, he also noted the patient had peripheral edema, jugular venous distension, and had spit up some pink-colored sputum into a cup by his bedside. These clues, all obtained within the first minute of our encounter, suggested a cardiac cause. So Jerry administered oxygen and asked the patient, 'Do you also have a history of heart problems?'

" 'Yeah, that tooooo . . . ' the patient struggled. 'Got so tired (gasp) of running to the bathroom to urinate (gasp) . . . that I stopped my (gasp) water pills, the Lasix, three days ago . . . (gasp) I'm gettin' worse by the hour. . . .' "

I could see the point Christenson was trying to make. The history pointed *more* to CHF than COPD, as originally suspected. The value of the second phase, the physical assessment, of the 60-Second Respiratory Exam became evident as Mark recounted the rest of the story.

"At that point," continued the car buff, "Jerry listened to the patient's chest. He heard good air exchange, but there were end-inspiratory rales at both bases. Putting the whole case together—the patient's stopping his water pills, the pinkish sputum, and the inspiratory rales—Jerry reasoned the patient's respiratory distress was caused by CHF."

"Did he treat the patient at that point?" I was anxious to know.

"Absolutely," confirmed Christenson. "Donnelly sat the patient upright, increased the oxygen to 90% by mask, gave sublingual nitro, pushed 80 mg of Lasix, and then loaded him for transport. After rechecking vitals, he repeated 0.4 mg sublingual nitro every 5 minutes en route."

"Did you guys get a good result?" I asked.

"Perfect," Mark beamed. "Within 10 minutes, we had a new patient on our hands. The man's respiratory rate had come down to 24 per minute, the heart rate had slowed to 100, and his skin had "pinked up." By the time we got to the hospital, the emergency department staff asked us why we had brought the patient in. Of course, that's typical with successful treatment of pulmonary edema. These patients can be almost gone one minute and ready to boogie a few minutes later. It's a very satisfying condition to treat if you've made the appropriate assessment.

"I asked Jerry why he didn't give the patient morphine. He said that he tries to avoid giving morphine to patients who have a history of significant COPD. Morphine tends to decrease respiratory drive in those patients. If the nitro and Lasix are ineffective, morphine can be considered."

Donnelly's two-step approach in the 60-Second Respiratory Assessment made a lot of sense to me.

"Let me see if I understand," I said in an attempt to clarify the 60-second strategy. "When it becomes necessary in the field to distinguish between cardiac and pulmonary causes for respiratory distress, the 60-second approach relies, first, on the past medical history as an initial guide—a beacon, of sorts—to suggest either CHF or COPD as the underlying cause. This initial assessment, which is usually based on the history alone, is then confirmed with the physical exam."

"You're getting the hang of it," Mark encouraged. "Now, what if the patient's history suggests both cardiac and pulmonary disease?"

I thought for a moment and then responded, "In patients who have a past history of *both* CHF and COPD, the EMT has to rely on the physical assessment to help discriminate between the two. In addition, he or she should try to elicit any history of recent changes in medication usage, especially discontinuation or noncompliance, and inquire about the presence of accompanying symptoms such as chest pain, syncope, or nausea and vomiting. These data will usually point the EMT in the right direction."

"You're going to be a 60-Second EMT in no time." Mark soaped up the hubcaps and whitewalls. "Let me tell you about one more case that will underscore what you just said. Two weeks ago, Jerry and I were called to see a 65-year-old man in acute respiratory distress. The guy had a history of both COPD and CHF. When we arrived, the patient's respiratory rate was 28, the heart rate was 120, and his skin was pink and dry.''

"Sounds like Donnelly had to decide between treatment for COPD or CHF,'' I offered. "The classic challenge.''

"It surely was,'' agreed Christenson. "But in this case, like the other, Jerry's 60-second history turned up some important clues. We learned the patient's steroid medications given to treat his COPD had recently been tapered off and that his aminophylline dosage had been cut in half by his private physician. That's enough to make any COPD decompensate, so, naturally, we leaned toward COPD as the cause for the patient's distress.''

> If patients have symptoms of both COPD and CHF, treatment with albuterol, nitro, and furosemide (Lasix) is appropriate.

"What else pushed you in that direction?'' I was curious to know.

"Well, on physical exam, the patient's breath sounds were markedly reduced in both lung fields, and there wasn't a crackle to be heard,'' Mark pointed out. "This was more evidence against congestive heart failure. Jerry used these additional historical data and the lack of inspiratory rales on physical exam to support his suspicion that the patient's distress was caused by chronic obstructive pulmonary disease rather than congestive heart failure.''

"Did Donnelly treat him for COPD?'' I asked.

"Sure did,'' continued Mark. "Continuous nebulized albuterol inhalers. They worked like a charm. If these patients have symptoms of both COPD and CHF, treatment with albuterol, nitro, and furosemide (Lasix) is appropriate.''

"Sounds like a foolproof system to me,'' I said.

"You're jumping the gun. No system is glitch-free, not even the 60-Second Respiratory Exam,'' Christenson said with conviction. "You see, there are other very important—even life-threatening—causes of respiratory distress besides heart failure and COPD.''

"Does Donnelly incorporate them into his 60-second program?'' I wondered.

"Absolutely,'' Christenson reassured me. "You see, although heart failure and COPD are the two most common causes of respiratory distress and the most difficult to separate, the EMT also has to consider other precipitating conditions. Pneumonia, allergic reactions, sepsis, and GI bleeding are among the other important causes of respiratory distress.''

''What does the EMT look for as part of his 60-second assessment?'' I asked.

''Again, the history is important,'' stressed Mark. ''Pneumonia is suggested by the presence of fever, shaking chills, and sputum production. Sepsis is a toxic state that frequently appears as respiratory distress; shaking chills, high fever, and altered mental status are often associated with sepsis. Anemia can cause respiratory distress because oxygen delivery to the tissues is compromised. The patient experiences shortness of breath. In fact, severe anemia can also lead to congestive heart failure. Pale conjunctiva, tarry stools, and hypotension should suggest occult GI bleeding as the cause of respiratory distress.''

> Any external event or internal condition that compromises oxygen delivery to the tissues can cause shortness of breath and respiratory distress.

''So any external event or internal condition that compromises oxygen delivery to the tissues can cause shortness of breath and respiratory distress?''

''Precisely. That's why, once he's excluded the more common causes, the 60-Second EMT has to consider carbon monoxide poisoning, cyanide ingestion, and other toxic inhalants as possible causes for respiratory distress. Aspiration also has to be ruled out.''

What I had come up with after talking with Christenson was a handful of ''pearls.'' The 60-second exam had clarified the important underlying causes of respiratory distress in older people. Hoping there were still more clinical pearls to be had, I turned my attention to younger patients with respiratory distress.

''Does the 60-Second EMT have a strategy for dealing with respiratory distress in patients with asthma and hyperventilation?'' I asked.

''Asthma, in particular, is stressed in the 60-Second Respiratory Assessment,'' informed Christenson as he packed a jar of car wax and a chamois into the trunk. ''Asthma patients are usually their own best diagnosticians. They know how severe their present attack is. They can compare it to previous attacks. They can tell you if they've ever required intubation or if their medications have been altered. If they've needed intubation in the past, it's a good indication the patient could deteriorate rapidly. If the patient has

Rapid-Access 60-SECOND EMT Guidelines: Rapid-Sequence Intubation

On occasion, rapidly deteriorating patients who are *in extremis* will require rapid-sequence intubation. Determining which patients with severe, life-threatening asthma require rapid-sequence intubation mandates a careful clinical assessment. This procedure should be performed only by experienced physicians, in those patients who have clearly failed more aggressive pharmacologic measures aimed at relieving bronchospasm, and in whom more conservative intubation techniques have been unsuccessful. In particular, patients with severe respiratory distress who have mental status changes, impending exhaustion, significant hypoxemia, or progressively rising $PaCO_2$ should be considered candidates for invasive airway intervention and mechanical ventilation. The following section outlines an orderly, systematic approach for this procedure, the pharmacologic agents used to perform rapid-sequence intubation, and guidelines for initiating mechanical ventilation.

Rapid-sequence intubation (RSI) permits the emergency physician to quickly secure airway access in a controlled manner and to ensure full patient compliance with the lung ventilations that follow. It involves the induction of general anesthesia and neuromuscular blockade in order to permit optimal intubation in the "unfasted" patient, with maximal protection against aspiration of stomach contents. RSI assumes that the patient has a full stomach, that full resuscitation facilities are available, and that a surgical airway can be established if attempts at intubation fail.

Positive-pressure ventilation before RSI should be avoided if the patient is awake and breathing because it can cause vomiting and lead to aspiration of gastric contents. In the event that the paralyzed patient cannot be intubated during RSI, *the physician must be prepared to perform cricothyroidotomy, to provide the patient a surgical airway*. At least one secure IV line should be established. Continuous cardiac and pulse oximeter monitoring are essential once the decision to perform RSI is made. An end tidal CO_2 monitor may be helpful in confirming placement of the endotracheal tube in the patient with a palpable pulse and blood pressure.

Necessary equipment, including adequate suction, endotracheal tubes, stylet, laryngoscope with both straight and curved blades, cricothyroidotomy tray, and bag-valve-mask with 100% oxygen, should also be at the bedside. A complete knowledge of airway anatomy, pharmacology, and ability to establish a surgical airway (cricothyroidotomy) are necessary prerequisites for RSI, which can be divided into the following phases:

PHASE I: PREOXYGENATION/PREPARATION (3 TO 5 MINUTES BEFORE INTUBATION)

This phase includes preparation of the patient and securing the necessary equipment. Preparation involves placing the patient on 100% oxygen. Preoxygenation for five minutes is preferred, although the preoxygenation period can be shortened by having the conscious patient take three full breaths of 100% oxygen.

PHASE II: PREMEDICATION (2 TO 3 MINUTES BEFORE INTUBATION)

During this phase, patients are premedicated with lidocaine (1 mg per kg) and pancuronium or vecuronium (.01 to .02 mg per kg). The lidocaine is used to help prevent harmful reflex responses that cause hypertension, cardiac arrhythmias, and increased intracranial pressure. The pancuronium or vecuronium is used to prevent fasciculations after succinylcholine is administered. Atropine (.01 mg per kg) is recommended for pediatric patients and is used to prevent bradycardia.

PHASE III: GENERAL ANESTHESIA/PARALYSIS (1 MINUTE BEFORE INTUBATION)

General anesthesia is induced with either thiopental (4 mg per kg) rapid IV push, midazolam (.1 to .3 mg per kg) IV push, or ketamine (.5 to 1 mg per kg) IV push. As mentioned previously, some experts consider ketamine to be the preferred agent in patients with asthma and severe bronchospasm, as well as in patients with hypotension or hypovolemia. Immediately after giving one of these agents, administer succinylcholine (1 to 1.5 mg per kg) or vecuronium (.25 mg per kg). If vecuronium is used, the defasciculating agent employed in the premedication phase (pancuronium, vecuronium) is not necessary.

labored breathing, extreme fatigue, or cyanosis, it's time to begin aggressive therapy, and call for an ALS unit for transport. The key is to get this information within the first minute of contact and then ask the patient what makes him better."

"What do you mean?" I asked.

"I wish you could see how Jerry does it right on the spot," he added, taking a last, long look at his sparkling Corvette.

PHASE IV: INTUBATION

About 30 seconds after the administration of the neuromuscular blocker, spontaneous respiration will begin to cease. At that time, an assistant should apply pressure over the cricoid cartilage (Sellick maneuver) so as to occlude the esophagus. Monitor for adequacy of neuromuscular blockade, and, when the jaw and mandible are completely relaxed, intubate the trachea under direct visualization. The Sellick maneuver should be maintained until tube placement has been confirmed by auscultation and end tidal–CO_2 detector. Endotracheal tube placement should also be confirmed with a chest radiograph. After intubation, you may need to consider longer-acting sedation and/or paralysis. When using vecuronium, be sure to use a generous amount of induction agent to avoid waiting too long to achieve optimal intubating conditions. *Succinylcholine is the most reliable agent and leads to complete relaxation within thirty to sixty seconds.* It is also much shorter-acting than vecuronium; paralysis lasts only 5 to 7 minutes with succinylcholine and about 60 minutes with vecuronium.

PHASE V: MECHANICAL VENTILATION

A variety of mechanical ventilators can provide the mechanical work necessary for the patient in respiratory failure. With certain pulmonary conditions, such as bronchospasm or respiratory distress syndrome, high pulmonary inflation pressures may be necessary. Because of this, volume-cycled ventilators are preferred for patients with these conditions. The physiology of asthma is primarily airway obstruction, mostly during the expiratory phase. Therefore adequate time should be allowed for expiration to minimize air trapping. Increasing the I:E ratio (1:3 or greater) and decreasing the ventilatory rate would provide for longer expiratory times. The use of positive end expiratory pressure (PEEP) in asthma is controversial; one study suggests that PEEP is detrimental when there is severe airflow obstruction. If PEEP is used at all, it should be used cautiously, maintaining efforts to keep peak airway pressure below 50 cm H_2O so as to minimize the chance of barotrauma.

"Maybe you can talk me through it," I suggested.

"Be glad to. When people have asthma, Jerry asks them what kind of bronchodilators have helped break their attacks in the past. He always wants to know if they have responded to albuterol, Alupent, epinephrine, aminophylline, or terbutaline. He asks when their last dose of medication was taken. This is the kind of information he obtains immediately and uses as a guide for therapy.

Beta-Adrenergic Agonists for Asthma

AGENT	AVAILABLE FORMS	PHARMACOKINETICS (INHALED)		
		ONSET (MIN)	PEAK (MIN)	DURATION (HR)
NONSELECTIVE				
Epinephrine	I, SC	5–10*	20	1
Ephedrine	O	60†	120–210	3–5
BETA-SELECTIVE				
Isoproterenol	I, IV	5	5–10	1
BETA₂-SELECTIVE				
Isoetharine	I	1–5	5–15	1–4
Metaproterenol	I, O	5–15	30–60	2.5–6
Terbutaline	I, O, SC	5–30	60–90	3–6
Albuterol‡	I, O, IV§	5–15	30–120	3–6

*Pharmacokinetics for subcutaneous administration.
†Pharmacokinetics for oral administration.
‡Also named "salbutamol" in Europe.
§IV form currently not available in the United States.
I = Inhaled; IV = intravenous; O = oral; SC = subcutaneous.

Remember, there's a strong psychological component to asthma, so these patients need to be reassured.

There's a strong psychological component to asthma, so these patients need to be reassured.

"Most of these patients can be managed with nebulized albuterol (mouthpiece or mask). This treatment can be given continuously during transport. If it is unsuccessful, subcutaneous epinephrine or terbutaline (for patients over 40) may be added. For patients in severe distress in whom cardiac arrest is imminent, Jerry immediately administers subcutaneous epinephrine."

After Mark finished, I felt reassured. I was confident that the next time I encountered a patient with respiratory distress, I would be able to use the 60-second exam to help initiate appropriate therapy and support the patient.

"I should mention two more conditions," Mark said, as he began to put his towels and polish in the trunk. "Don't forget upper-airway obstruction caused by allergic reactions. That's a 60-second diagnosis if there ever was one. You usually don't have more than a minute to initiate treatment if you want to do any good. These patients can go down the tubes fast!"

"What's the 60-second key?"

"To establish that the respiratory distress has been caused by some allergic reaction," he said. "Ask if there's been a bee sting or insect bite, or if they've eaten anything that they may be allergic to. Look for mucous-membrane swelling in the mouth. Usually, there is inspiratory stridor, too."

"Treatment in these cases is epinephrine, oxygen, and Benadryl®, right?" I asked.

"That's right. If the patient is in severe distress and shock, you may need to give epinephrine 1:10000 IV. IV fluids are also appropriate since vasodilation and vessel permeability can cause profound hypotension."

"Well, I guess that about does it."

"Almost," Christenson said. "Don't forget that tricky group of patients with hyperventilation."

"Why do you call them 'tricky?' " I wanted to know.

"Because although they don't have any signs of respiratory distress—like cyanosis, wheezes, rales, or stridor—the metabolic changes caused by hyperventilation can result in syncope, delirium, agitation, carpopedal spasm, and, sometimes, seizures. These symptoms may confuse the picture.

"The key for these patients is reassurance. Avoid paper bags or O_2 masks with no oxygen flowing. If you make an assessment error, you can contribute to further hypoxia. A pulse oximeter may help with your assessment. **If in doubt, give oxygen!**"

By this time, Mark had nestled himself comfortably into the bucket seat of his car, put his seat belt on, and started the engine. It purred. In fact, it sounded as if it had rolled off the assembly line yesterday.

"Take care, now," he said, with a gleam in his eye.

Then he sped off before I could even say "Thanks."

Zany, yes. Brilliant, too. In fact, it was enough to take my breath away.

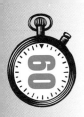

RESPIRATION

I. Previous History: Let the patient be your guide—a history of congestive heart failure or chronic obstructive pulmonary disease is a valuable clue as to the nature of the current episode, because either condition can frequently recur in the same patient.

   The list of the patient's current medications is also invaluable in establishing his or her medical history.

   A. CHF drugs: diuretics, digitalis derivatives, Amrinone® (Inocor®), nitrates (e.g., nitroglycerin ointment, isosorbide dinitrate), nifedipine, diltiazem (Cardizem®).

   B. COPD drugs: aminophylline, theophylline, and their many derivatives, metaproterenol, isoproterenol, albuterol, cromolyn, prednisone, dexamethasone inhalers, azamacort). Aminophylline and theophylline preparations are losing popularity because of high probabilities of toxicity.

II. Ask about events leading up to the current episode of dyspnea.

   A. Lack of compliance in taking maintenance medications for either CHF or COPD (see above) usually leads to exacerbation of the respective disease process.

   Any recent change in the medication history, whether it was caused by the patient's noncompliance, a nursing home error, or a physician's order, should alert you to potential worsening of the underlying process.

   B. Additional events leading to the exacerbation of CHF:

      1. Recent history of worsening of the following symptoms:

         a. Orthopnea: Has the patient had to sleep in a more upright position recently? Has he or she had to use more pillows in order to sleep the past night or two?

         b. Nocturnal dyspnea: Has the patient character-

istically been waking up in the middle of the night with shortness of breath? If yes, what has made the shortness of breath better?
   i. Improvement as a result of sitting up or going to the window to get fresh air is indicative of paroxysmal nocturnal dyspnea (PND), which suggests CHF.
   ii. Improvement of nocturnal dyspnea as a result of clearing the throat of mucous secretions is consistent with COPD.
  2. Worsening of ankle swelling also suggests CHF—especially if it is associated with one of the above events and if it is bilateral.

   If the ankle swelling is sudden, unilateral, and associated with pain, heat, and redness, you must consider thrombophlebitis, viewing the shortness of breath as a symptom of potential **pulmonary embolism**.

C. Additional events leading to the exacerbation of COPD:
  1. Recent history of increased cough and sputum production—especially if purulent or very bloody.
    Note: Frequently the patient complains of intense congestion in his or her chest but is unable to bring any sputum up.
  2. Pleuritic chest pain: Suspect complicating **spontaneous pneumothorax**.
  3. Exposure to environmental respiratory irritants on hot, humid days.
  4. Fever, especially in association with C-1.
  5. Pulmonary embolism (see above for CHF).

III. Physical Examination clues.
  A. The patient with CHF shows one or more of the following:
  1. He or she sits bolt upright.
  2. There may be a gurgling type of breathing and in *extreme* cases there is frothy pink sputum in the mouth or pharynx.

3. There may be a regular alternation of the strength in the patient's pulse despite a regular sinus tachycardia. This is called pulsus alternans.

4. There is jugular venous distension if the patient has a thin enough neck to allow you to see it. Occasionally, this JVD becomes more prominent if you put constant, firm pressure over the right upper quadrant of the patient's abdomen (this is called hepatojugular reflux).

5. There is ankle edema that pits when you put prolonged pressure into the ankle.

6. When you examine the chest, you hear moist late inspiratory crackles (rales) at the base of both lungs—or all over the lung fields if the CHF is bad enough.

Unilateral crackles from CHF are usually on the right side and are almost always heard in the dependent portions of the patient's lungs (water settles).

B. The patient with COPD can be described by one or more of the following:

1. He or she might have the body habitus of either a "pink puffer" or a "blue bloater."

2. He or she sits upright.

3. There is often pursed-lip breathing.

4. When you examine the chest you frequently note the following:

a. Poor air movement—occasionally you barely hear any air movement.

b. If your patient is moving enough air, you hear coarse rhonchi—usually on expiration—occasionally in association with wheezes throughout the chest.

Remember that pneumonia can produce very localized crackles anywhere in the chest, regardless of which part is dependent.

c. If breath sounds are asymmetric (decreased on one side), percuss the chest:

i. If one side is abnormally flat to percussion, there is probably an effusion.

       ii. If one side is abnormally hollow (shows increased resonance), suspect pneumothorax.

IV. Never forget the possibility of **Upper-Airway Obstruction**. Suspect this when:

  A. The history is suggestive (i.e., upper-airway trauma, recent food or foreign-body ingestion, swelling of the mouth or pharynx).

  B. Massive use of the accessory muscles of respiration occurs with very poor to no movement of air from the mouth.

  C. Drooling occurs.

  D. Difficulty with *inspiration* over expiration, especially if there is inspiratory *stridor*—noisy, wheezy sounds on inspiration.

V. **Asthma** is a frequent cause of respiratory distress, especially in younger patients.

  A. These patients are frequently their own best diagnosticians.

  B. Ask asthma patients what precipitated the current attack; how the current attack compares in severity to past attacks; whether or not they have had to be intubated in the past, and what they have done for their attacks.

  C. The duration of the current attack is important: the longer the duration of the attack, the more difficult it is to "break" it.

  D. Any asthmatic currently taking prednisone cannot be easily treated and probably should be hospitalized.

  E. Especially dangerous signs in the asthmatic:

    1. Cyanosis: This occurs only very late in the pure asthmatic.

    2. Drowsiness and/or extreme fatigue: This implies CO_2 retention, again a late sign.

    3. Stridor: When this occurs, suspect laryngospasm, which may eventually require a surgical airway.

    4. Pulsus paradoxicus: In taking your patient's

blood pressure, see if you lose the top level of systolic sounds on inspiration. If you do, your patient has a paradoxical pulse. If the range of systolic pressure in which this occurs is over 20 mm Hg, this is a significant pulsus paradoxicus, which signifies a severe attack.

Remember that a paradoxical pulse can occur in other clinical conditions, including cardiac tamponade. Consider the clinical context.

    5. No wheezing and barely audible breath sounds may imply *severe* bronchospasm.

F. Patients with a long history of persistent asthma should be treated for all intents and purposes like COPD patients—especially with regard to administering low-flow O_2.

VI. **60-Second Triage**

A. Respiratory distress is usually an **ALS** call.

B. **BLS** transport can probably be accomplished in rare circumstances such as:

    1. A mild exacerbation of known asthma in a patient who has minimal respiratory distress.

    2. Clear-cut hyperventilation syndrome in a young patient, especially if there is a prior history of the same.

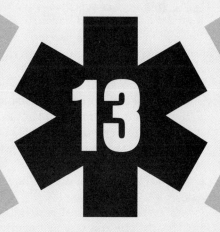

13

The 60-Second Assessment of Thermoregulatory Disorders

y watch told me that it was 5:00 AM. I had been up for four hours! Hal Weisser and I had left town at 1:00 AM for our "meeting" and had arrived at Timberline Lodge at 3:00 AM. We had been climbing the side of a rock for almost two hours.

Hal was an avid outdoorsman and was active in Oregon Mountain Rescue. His area of interest was environmental emergencies and heat illness.

I had met Hal at an in-service on hypothermia that he and Jerry had given. I told him that I wanted to learn more about heat emergencies and the 60-Second EMT. He smiled and suggested we get together that weekend for our meeting, which turned out to be a climbing trip on Mount Hood. "What better way to learn more about environmental illness than out in the environment?" he asked.

We stopped for a rest and Hal politely waited for me to catch my breath. The sun was just coming up over White River Canyon and we began to take in the beautiful view.

"Humans must maintain a narrow range of temperature to function properly. Their thermoregulatory mechanisms maintain stable body temperature within a very narrow range despite changing environments and changing metabolic needs. Extremes in body temperature require rapid recognition and intervention."

I was shivering from the wind and cool air and from sitting on snow. I told Hal that being cold seemed to be something I could relate to.

"That's true," Hal said, "but hypothermia, or reduced core temperature, is not unique to very cold environments. We all recognize immersion in cold water, or being lost in a snowstorm as high-risk situations for hypothermia. But the risk is often much more subtle. As with many illnesses, people at the extremes of age are the most susceptible. Small children have a higher surface area to body mass–ratio than adults and therefore lose heat more quickly.

Small children have a higher surface area to body mass–ratio than adults and therefore lose heat more quickly.

"Geriatric patients and adults with underlying illness and low reserves get into trouble much more quickly also. People at extreme ages are less able to carry out adaptive activities to maintain body temperature, as are adults with altered level of consciousness. Drug and alcohol users are also more susceptible."

"What are the main causes of hypothermia?" I asked through chattering teeth.

"Causes of hypothermia fall into three main categories. Increased heat loss, such as results from exposure in a cold environment, is the most familiar. In cold, dry environments heat is lost through skin and breathing. With wet clothes or immersion in cold water, heat loss increases 5 to 25 times as rapidly, respectively, for given ambient temperature. Hypothermia can occur in relatively warm temperatures by these mechanisms."

With wet clothes or immersion in cold water, heat loss increases 5 to 25 times as rapidly, respectively, for given ambient temperature.

Hal went on, "Heat loss through skin is increased if there is significant loss of intact skin. Burn patients are very susceptible to heat loss. Vasodilation of superficial blood vessels from medications and, especially, alcohol leads to increased heat loss. A common scenario is played out when a person becomes intoxicated during the afternoon, passes out outside in the cool evening or night, and becomes hypothermic. Another cause of increased heat loss is rapid administration of large amounts of cold IV solution during resuscitation."

I remembered that this had been a problem with trauma patients in long transport before heated solutions became available.

"What about the other causes?" I prompted.

"Decreased heat production is the second major category leading to hypothermia. Endocrine disorders of the pituitary, thyroid, or adrenal glands cause deficiency of stress hormones and reduce the ability to regulate temperature and generate heat. History of endocrine disease should be obtained in all cases of hypothermia. Diabetes, because of reduced glucose and body stores of glycogen,

Diabetes can increase susceptibility to hypothermia.

can increase susceptibility to hypothermia. Starvation from malnutrition or prolonged exertion also augments susceptibility to hypothermia."

Hal's remark reminded me that it was time to eat something.

Hal agreed. "It's 20 degrees with a breeze and we're burning a lot of calories per hour while climbing." He continued his lesson as I searched the backpack for something edible.

"Impaired ability to regulate temperature is the third major category. Central failure implies loss of CNS control of thermoregulation. Head injury, strokes, drug overdoses, and Parkinson's disease all are associated with increased risk of hypothermia probably related to deficiency in centrally controlled vasoconstriction. Cerebellar disease can lead to hypothermia in cold environments because of inadequate or uncoordinated shivering.

"Peripheral nerve disorders, spinal cord injury, and diabetes interfere with neural control of peripheral vasodilation and increase susceptibility to cold environments." Hal smiled as I pulled my parka out of the pack.

"Can you give me an example?"

"Sure. A small child playing outside on a cold winter afternoon as his clothes become soaked by snow, the sun goes down, and the temperature drops or an elderly person who has fallen with a hip fracture would not be able to carry out the most basic adaptation or regulation of their environment." I nodded in understanding.

"Hypothermia is categorized into mild, moderate, and severe forms. Mild hypothermia is defined as a core temperature of 34 degrees centigrade (93.2°F) to normal temperature. In otherwise healthy individuals, thermogenesis is at a maximum in this range. An increase in metabolic rate and maximal shivering occurs as core temperatures drops. Speech becomes slurred and incoordination develops. Geriatric patients can become very apathetic and confused. A flat affect, altered level of consciousness, or decreased functioning may be the only history that is available in this age group."

We got up at this point and continued up the gentle slope. "We'll stop at Illumination Saddle and continue our discussion," he said. I realized that our discussion had become a monologue as I concentrated on my climbing and breathing while Hal talked on.

"In moderate hypothermia, that is, 30 degrees centigrade (86.0°F), cardiac irritability appears. Atrial fibrillation and, with lower temperatures, ventricular fibrillation are common. Metabolic activity decreases, shivering stops, and victims are not able to generate sufficient heat to warm themselves. Stupor and coma ensue. Many pharmacologic agents lose effectiveness in this temperature range. Insulin becomes ineffective and pressor agents such as dopamine and dobutamine are much less effective at lower temperatures because of reduced activity at the tissue level and the fact that maximum vasoconstriction has already occurred. Not only are they not beneficial in increasing pressure, but dysrhythmic side effects persist."

I had often wondered why aggressive drug therapy was discouraged in cases of hypothermia.

"Many drugs lose effectiveness at lower temperatures. You can overdose. Repeating medications that are not effective and not metabolized can result in toxic concentrations when rewarming of a patient is achieved."

"Severe hypothermia is defined as 30 degrees centigrade (86.0°F) and less. Coma ensues and profound hypotension, decreased respirations, and, ultimately, apnea develop. Ventricular fibrillation risk increases, or bradycardia degenerates to asystole as the temperature drops."

"Treatment begins with recognition. If we found someone facedown in the snow it would be obvious. When the call is for an 82-year-old with altered level of consciousness, the diagnosis is more difficult. Prevention of further heat loss is paramount. Transferring the patient from the cold environment and removing any wet clothing is the first treatment. Heated, humidified O_2, if available, is the safest of rewarming methods

> Treatment begins with recognition. Prevention of further heat loss is paramount.

and should be used for all levels of hypothermia. Treatments for warming the extremities, such as heated blankets or hot tub soaks, run the risk that peripheral vasodilation might cause very cold blood to reenter the circulation and further lower the core temperature, thus worsening the symptoms.

"Hypotension, bradycardia, and decreased respirations occur in severe hypothemia. Careful assessment is needed to differentiate a true cardiac arrest from a greatly reduced output. In prolonged hypothermia with peripheral vasoconstriction, blood is shunted to the core causing a central hypervolemia. A cold diuresis ensues from the central fluid overload and from the reduced renal ability

Clinical Signs and Symptoms of Hypothermia

CLASS	CORE TEMPERATURE °C	CORE TEMPERATURE °F	SIGNS AND SYMPTOMS
Mild	36°	96.8°	Increased metabolic rate, maximum shivering
Moderate	34°	93.2°	Impaired judgment, slurred speech
	30°	86.0°	Respiratory depression, myocardial irritability, bradycardia, atrial fibrillation, decreased metabolic activity
Severe	<30°	<86.0°	Coma, profound hypotension, decreased respirations, fixed and dilated pupils, spontaneous ventricular fibrillation

to concentrate urine. Rewarming and increasing peripheral circulation can lead to profound hypotension if there has been a significant cold diuresis. If pulmonary edema is not also present because of central overload, a fluid challenge should be given.

"Ventricular fibrillation threshold is greatly lowered in severe hypothermia. Handling and transport must be as gentle as possible. Shallow respirations and bradycardia can be tolerated with a decreased metabolic demand. In hypothermia patients, intubation, drug therapy, and CPR should be reserved for true arrests."

"What are the patient's chances of survival in these cases?"

"Survival has been reported after prolonged submersion, with hypothermia, protracted asystole, and core temperatures as low as 16 degrees centigrade. This confirms the adage 'No one is dead until he is warm and dead.' "

After this exposition of cold illness, which I had interrupted very little because of my tachypnea, we stopped at Illumination Saddle. We needed to eat again and then put on harness, rope, and our crampons for the short glacier traverse and the steep couloir at the head of the Reid glacier.

The wind had died down and the sun was very warm, even though the air was still cool. With my heavy clothes and the exertion of climbing, I had become quite warm.

"I think I've talked enough about hypothermia," said Hal. "You've generated so much heat coming up this last slope, maybe we should talk about hyperthermia. Just as a person does not have to be in freezing temperature to become hypothermic, he does not have to be in 100-degree temperature to have hyperthermia."

"So what does cause hyperthermia?" I asked as I trudged behind him.

Hyperthermia, or elevated core temperature, occurs when an external/internal heat load exceeds the body's capacity to dissipate the heat.

"Hyperthermia, or elevated core temperature, occurs when an external/internal heat load exceeds the body's capacity to dissipate the heat. Resting normal body metabolism would raise body temperature 1.1 degrees centigrade in an hour without mechanisms to dissipate heat. Heavy exercise can increase heat generation up to five times. This amount of heat loss is accomplished in only two ways: (1) Transfer of heat from a warm body to a cool environment (this mechanism ceases as ambient temperature approaches or exceeds body temperature), or (2) evaporative cooling of sweat, which is the only physiologic heat-loss mechanism in environmental temperatures roughly 34 degrees centigrade (93°F) or higher.''

"Go on," I nodded.

"As with hypothermia, exposure to extreme environments is an obvious cause but not a requirement for development of heat illness. Again, people at the extremes of age are most susceptible, and many different conditions can lead to hyperthermia.

"Heat loss by conduction to the environment is a fixed quantity dependent only on ambient temperature. Evaporative cooling by peripheral vasodilation and sweating is the body's only controllable heat-loss mechanism. Any condition that affects this mechanism of evaporative cooling will predispose a person to heat illness. Underlying heart disease decreases heat tolerance because the heart may not maintain adequate output with peripheral vasodilation. Dehydration, from any cause, decreases sweating and reduces ability to dissipate heat. Drugs with anticholinergic effect, such as antihistamines, antidepressants, and antipsychotic medications, act to decrease sweating and increase the risk of hyperthermia.

> Dehydration, from any cause, decreases sweating and reduces ability to dissipate heat.

"Increased heat production can occur for many reasons; infection is the most common. Heavy exercise, even in healthy adults, can produce heat more rapidly than it is lost through normal mechanisms. Stimulant drugs, such as PCP, amphetamines, or LSD, that produce hyperactivity and muscle rigidity can lead to high core temperatures. Rigidity and tremulousness from alcohol withdrawal can also cause these.''

At this point we dropped down from the Saddle and began the short traverse to the couloir that would take us to the summit. As we started up, I was grateful that the steps Hal kicked in the snow held my weight. He slowed his pace so that I could climb the steep slope without gasping for breath. The exertion dried my mouth and I knew our conversation would again become Hal's monologue.

"In hypothermia, below 30 degrees centigrade (86°F), effective heat production is lost. Similarly, in hyperthermia there are minor syndromes in which thermoregulatory mechanisms are maintained.

"Minor syndromes include heat edema of hands and feet, prickly heat, and heat cramps from vasodilation. Prickly heat is an extremely pruritic rash caused by plugging of the sweat glands, which occurs in hot, humid environments. Heat cramps trouble a person during heavy exertion; they respond to rest or moving to a cooler environment and stretching. An oral salt solution or IV normal saline can also be helpful. All of these syndromes can occur with a normal body temperature."

Hal, not even short of breath, continued. "More severe is heat exhaustion. This generally develops over an extended period of time—many hours or days. With peripheral vasodilation, prolonged increased cardiac work is needed to maintain a normal temperature. Dehydration, if present, can produce symptoms of malaise, fatigue, anorexia, nausea, vomiting, thirst, and weakness. Mental status remains intact, though irritability or anxiety may be present. Temperature is maintained at normal, or only 1 to 2 degrees higher than normal, and sweating may or may not be present. After evaluation of orthostatics and assessment of dehydration, establish IV, challenge with normal saline fluid, and transport the patient."

> Heat exhaustion generally develops over an extended period of time.

"How are heat exhaustion and heat stroke different?"

"A heat stroke includes all the symptoms of heat exhaustion; but also the ability to regulate temperature is lost, which leads to markedly elevated core temperature. Mental-status changes occur, including obtundation, coma, seizures, and, ultimately, death. Cellular damage and CNS damage take place extremely rapidly at core temperatures above 41 degrees centigrade (105.8°F), aggressive treatment is critical.

"Airway protection with endotracheal intubation is needed if seizures or coma are present. Dehydration may not be present if hyperthermia has occurred over a short period of time—for example, if a small child has been left in a hot car, a foundry worker has become overheated, or someone has passed out in a steam bath. However, the more typical presentation is an elderly individual, a young child, or an impaired adult who has been exposed to prolonged heat stress."

> Evaporative cooling is by far the most effective and safest heat-loss mechanism.

"What should EMTs do when they encounter patients experiencing heat stress?"

"Rapid cooling should be started immediately. Remove all clothing and remove the patient from the heat source. Ice packs should be placed in the axilla and groin areas. Large blood flows in these areas will help facilitate heat loss. The victim should be wet down and fanned. Evaporative cooling is by far the most effective and safest heat-loss mechanism. Very cold water, or ice-water, baths are less effective; rapid skin cooling can lead to vasoconstriction, which reduces blood flow to the periphery where it can be available for heat exchange. This can lead to shivering, which generates *more* heat and raises the core temperature.''

"Defeating the purpose," I mused.

"Exactly!" Hal confirmed.

By now, we found ourselves on the last part of the summit ridge. Hal coiled the rope as I slowly traversed the ridge over the steep North Face. Making the last rise in the ridge, I could see what was left of Mount Saint Helens, and off in the distance I saw Mount Adams and Mount Rainier. A sense of exhilaration overwhelmed me as I realized that I had expanded my mind as well as my horizons.

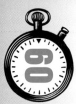

ASSESSING THERMOREGULATORY DISORDER

HYPOTHERMIA

(1) Rare in healthy adults except in extreme environments.
(2) Occurs in the elderly and infants much more readily.
(3) Possible underlying causes to consider:
   (a) Endocrine disease.
   (b) Alcohol and alcoholism, drug ingestion.
   (c) CNS disorders.
(4) Treatment:
   (a) Warmed humidified O_2.
   (b) Gentle handling.
   (c) Treatment with fluid challenge if blood pressure is low.
   (d) Caution with cardioactive drugs.
   (e) Prolonged resuscitation efforts, which can be successful.

HYPERTHERMIA

(1) Occurs in the elderly and infants more readily.
(2) Possible underlying causes to consider:
   (a) Heart disease.
   (b) Many drugs and medications.
(3) Treatment:
   (a) For heat stroke, airway protection.
   (b) Aggressive cooling, ice packs to groin and axilla.
   (c) Wet towels or mist and fanning.
   (d) Slowing down cooling if shivering develops.

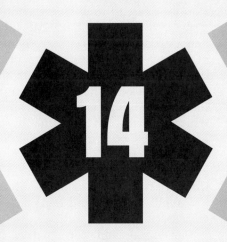

The 60–Second
Neurologic Exam

aren Brooks was one of the most active EMTs in Donnelly's regional EMS system. She was politically aware and a strong advocate of EMT rights. Karen was a vocal proponent of improved salary scales, benefit packages, and working conditions that were in keeping with the increasing professional responsibilities that have been assumed by prehospital providers. She was acutely aware of critical-incident stress and burnout, from which so many EMTs eventually suffer. Karen led a small group of EMT leaders to reform schedules, upgrade continuing-education funds, and improve vacation benefits offered by the private ambulance company for which she worked. Brooks had made extraordinary progress fighting a system that seemed insensitive to the plight of EMTs and their lack of job security and salary increases.

Developing and participating in continuing-education programs were a critical part of the campaign she waged against burnout among EMTs. Jerry Donnelly had been one of the instructors asked to participate in her teaching seminars. Brooks was especially interested in neurologic assessment and, along with Donnelly, had developed a 60-Second Neurologic Exam that was praised throughout the region.

I met Brooks at the Satellite Grill, a real down-home diner. It had a reputation among EMTs for great buttermilk pancakes, fresh pies, and other old-fashioned American dishes.

"Karen, hello. Thanks for meeting me on such short notice," I said, as I shook her hand and nestled myself into a banquette made of pink Naugahyde. She was drinking a chocolate egg cream. I flagged down a waitress and pointed to Brooks's drink, indicating that I wanted one also.

"No problem," Karen answered. "I'm always willing to participate in any activity that will improve the clinical skills of EMTs. You know, after we finished talking on the phone last night, I thought for a while about how Donnelly has earned his reputation as the 60-Second EMT."

She paused, sipped her drink, then said "That *is* what you want to know, isn't it?"

"That's exactly what I want to know," I said.

"Well, there are so many things about Jerry," she continued, "but the one aspect of his 60-second system that stands out is the 60-Second Neurologic Exam."

"Great! I'd like to hear more about it." The waitress set my egg cream on the table.

"The critical thing about Donnelly's 60-Second Neuro Assessment," Brooks began, "is that it can be used in so many different clinical situations, from multiple trauma to geriatric medicine. A wide range of clinical disorders, from infection and metabolic disorders to myocardial infarction and hypertensive cerebrovascular disease, have presenting neurologic signs and symptoms."

Karen's point was well taken. EMTs who are able to accurately assess neurologic signs and symptoms are usually ahead of the game pinning down the underlying cause of a patient's problem. For example, EMTs who recognize that the sudden onset of delirium, confusion, and headache in a patient with hypertension can be the first sign of a subarachnoid hemorrhage most likely make appropriate triage decisions and transport the patient to a facility equipped to treat neurosurgical emergencies. Prehospital care providers who know how to recognize focal neurologic deficits are one critical step closer to sifting out possible causes of the problem, whether it be atrial fibrillation or hyper-

> Prehospital care providers who know how to recognize focal neurologic deficits are one critical step closer to sifting out possible causes of the problem.

Physical Findings Suggestive of Specific Stroke Syndromes

CAROTID TIA
Hemiparesis or monoparesis
Hemiparesthesia or monohypesthesia
Hemihypesthesia or monohypesthesia
Aphasia
Monocular visual loss (amaurosis fugax)
Homonymous hemianopia
Combination of the above

VERTEBROBASILAR TIA
Monoparesis, hemiparesis, or quadriparesis
Paresthesia, hypesthesia, in various combinations over one or both
   sides of the body or face
Loss of vision, bilateral or unilateral homonymous hemianopsia
Ataxia
Hearing loss, unilateral or bilateral
Combination of the above

---

osmolar coma associated with adult-onset diabetes. The 60-Second Neuro Exam can be the linchpin in assessing a wide variety of common clinical disorders.

The 60-Second Neuro Exam is a ten-point exam that's tailor-made for rapid prehospital assessment of the neurologically impaired patient.

"You know that the docs use laboratory tests, CAT scans, and MRIs to diagnose neurologic disorders in the hospital setting," Brooks mused. "Obviously, we don't have these procedures available to us in the field. Yet we come very close to making the correct assessment simply by using the 60-Second Neuro Exam."

"Is the 60-Second Neuro Exam a modification of the Glasgow Coma Scale?" I asked.

"Not at all," Karen informed. "It's a ten-point exam that's tailor-made for rapid prehospital assessment of the neurologically impaired patient."

"Why don't you take me through it?" I suggested.

"That's what we're here for." She smiled and began to outline a unique assessment strategy. "The ten parts of the 60-Second EMT Neurologic Exam include:

(1) Mental status and LOC
(2) Speech
(3) Meninges
(4) Skull and spine
(5) Station and gait
(6) The twelve cranial nerves
(7) Motor function
(8) Sensory function
(9) Cerebellar function
(10) Deep tendon reflexes

A skilled EMT can finish this exam in less than a minute if she is systematic."

"Is this ten-point assessment complete enough to pinpoint the cause of a patient's problem in the field?" I asked.

"If you want to know the truth, it's actually more comprehensive than most neuro exams you see physicians doing in the emergency department," she answered. "The nice thing is that each component of the 60-Second Neuro Exam leads the EMT to a specific diagnosis or clinical disorder."

"I think it would help me if you took me through the ten-point exam and pointed out the correlations between physical findings and clinical states,'' I offered.

''That's what I came prepared to do,'' Brooks said as she signaled to the waitress that she wanted a refill on her chocolate egg cream. ''Let's go through Donnelly's exam, point by point. The patient's mental status, the first component of the 60-Second Approach to Neurologic Assessment, is key. EMTs must always assume that a patient's baseline mental status is normal and treat him or her on that basis. This is true even for elderly patients and alcoholics. I've seen too many EMTs ascribe mental confusion in an elderly patient to advanced age when, in fact, there was something much more serious going on: a drug reaction, a subdural hematoma, or a severe metabolic disorder. When you are treating patients who have sustained head trauma while under the influence of alcohol, it is safe for purposes of triage to assume that the impaired mental status has been caused by something other than the intoxicant. You may end up treating the patient too aggressively but that's better than missing a life-threatening problem.''

''What are the key components of a mental status exam in Donnelly's system?'' I asked.

''First, assess how oriented the patient is to time, place, and person,'' Brooks explained. ''If any one of these is deficient, a significant underlying problem is present. Note also the content of the patient's thought patterns. If the patient isn't making sense, is having a difficult time following a train of thought, has recent memory loss, has perceptual disturbances, or is hallucinating, the EMT is probably dealing with a global derangement of consciousness, in other words, delirium. Delirium, which is also referred to as an acute confusional state, is characterized by impairment of higher mental functions in a patient who shows clouding of consciousness.''

> **Always assume that a patient's baseline mental status is normal and treat him or her on that basis.**

''And what's the importance of recognizing delirium?''

''It is crucial because delirium reflects a widespread dysfunction in brain tissue that is frequently caused by disease processes outside the central nervous system,'' Brooks explained. ''For example, strange behavior at night, wandering, disorientation, or restlessness, combined with periods of memory loss and confusion, personality change, and a recent physical illness. A cold which has turned into a pneumonia

Types of Delirium	
"NOISY"	**"QUIET"**
Restlessness	Drowsiness
Agitation	Lethargy
Fear	Poor concentration
Anxiety	Distractibility
Illusion	
Hallucinations	

is one of the common presentations of delirium in the prehospital setting. The importance of recognizing delirium can hardly be overemphasized since it is a more common early symptom of physical illness in the older patient than fever, pain, or tachycardia."

"I've heard EMTs describe so-called delirious patients," I remarked, "but the strange thing is, their descriptions varied widely. Are there different kinds of delirium the 60-Second EMT should learn to recognize?"

"In fact, there are," Karen said. "They are commonly called 'noisy' and 'quiet' forms of delirium. The noisy form, which is marked by restlessness, agitation, fear, anxiety, illusions, and hallucinations, is usually associated with alcohol or drug intoxication, but it may occur with any illness. The so-called quiet form of delirium is more common among the elderly and is characterized by drowsiness, lethargy, poor concentration, and distractibility. Some people alternate between the two forms. It's important to know that, frequently, the first symptom of Alzheimer's disease is delirium that's been triggered by a seemingly trivial event."

Frequently, the first symptom of Alzheimer's disease is delirium that's been triggered by a seemingly trivial event.

"So what should go through the 60-Second EMT's mind when he encounters a delirious patient?"

"That's not an easy question to answer, because an enormous variety of physical illnesses can cause delirium. Realizing the importance of trying to narrow down these possibilities for his EMTs, Donnelly created a mnemonic for disorders caused by delirium."

"Oh, yeah? What is it?"

"MADCAP," Brooks announced.

"You've got to be kidding!"

Remember MADCAP

M for Medication reactions and Metabolic derangements (e.g., hypoglycemia).
A for Alcohol and Anticholinergics
D for Dementia.
C for Cardiac disorders and Cerebrovascular accident (CVA).
A for Alterations in hemodynamic or respiratory status.
P for Pneumonia and associated sepsis.

"As a matter of fact, I'm not," she said. "The **M** stands for **M**edication reactions and **M**etabolic disturbances such as dehydration, and hypo- and hyperglycemia. **A** is a reminder that **A**lcohol is a common cause of delirium in the young and middle-aged groups, and that **A**nticholinergic syndromes are prevalent in the elderly. The **D** stands for **D**ementia, including Alzheimer's, which, in the geriatric age group, first may be found by the EMT as delirium."

"Sounds good so far," I said. "Continue."

The **C** in MADCAP represents **C**ardiac and **C**erebrovascular disorders, such as stroke, intracerebral hemorrhage, subarachnoid hemorrhage, chronic subdural hematoma, and myocardial infarction. The second **A** in MADCAP stands for **A**lterations in hemodynamic and respiratory status, as well as alterations in the patient's environment, which can precipitate a delirious state. The **P** stands for **P**neumonia and other underlying infections that commonly produce delirium in susceptible age groups, particularly, the elderly."

The MADCAP mnemonic hit the nail right on the head when it came to teasing out the illnesses associated with delirium.

"Are there some specific drugs or conditions that immediately go through Donnelly's mind when he encounters a patient with altered mental status?" I inquired.

"The MADCAP approach covers most of them, but I can be more specific," Brooks replied. "In general, cardiovascular conditions, infections, and drugs are responsible for the majority of delirious states in the elderly. Congestive heart failure, myocardial infarction, various arrhythmias, pneumonia, chronic respiratory disease, and urinary infections, as well as major strokes are among the more important causes. As far as drugs are concerned, digitalis, steroids, antihypertensive agents (especially diuretics and beta blockers), salicylates, oral hypoglycemics, tricyclic antidepressants, antidepressants, and benzodiazepines may all produce delirious states. Also, dehydration and electrolyte disturbances, hypothermia, cancer, and severe pain caused by herpes zoster, glaucoma, a toothache, or fecal impaction may cause confusional states, particularly if dementia is already present."

> **The EMT should recognize speech disorders, especially aphasia.**

"Karen, that's the best approach I've heard yet for getting to the bottom of confusional states," I said. "And that's only the first component of the neuro exam, right?"

"That's right," she replied. "Now, as far as coma goes, I'm sure Jerry has told you he developed a special module."

"He did, and, as a matter of fact, I met Frank Zimmer, who took me through the 60-Second Coma Exam."

"Good, so let's go on to speech function, the second component of the 60-Second Neuro Exam. The EMT should recognize speech disorders, especially aphasia. If a patient is relatively alert but isn't able to understand simple verbal commands, he has what's called a *receptive* aphasia. An *expressive* aphasia is characterized by inappropriate word choices and nonsensical sentences. This is called Wernicke's aphasia. If a patient has this problem, suspect stroke as an underlying cause."

"What about slurring of words?" I asked.

"That's a little different. If the words and sentences all make sense, but the words sound fuzzy, the patient may have a dysarthria," Brooks explained. "Dysarthria is caused by brainstem lesions that prevent the patient from pronouncing words correctly."

"That sounds straightforward," I commented.

"It is," the EMT said. "Now let's go on to the meninges. Of course, the 60-Second EMT should never test for meningeal irritation when trauma is involved. C-spine stabilization is indicated in those situations. In examining the medical patient, though, the EMT can gently lift the patient's head. Detected stiffness or pain with movement is a good indication that meningeal irritation is present."

> **Usually the underlying cause of meningeal irritation is infectious meningitis, subarachnoid hemorrhage, or some other inflammatory condition.**

"What does meningeal irritation suggest?"

"It means there is an inflammatory process involving the meningeal layer of the brain," explained Brooks. "Usually the underlying cause of meningeal irritation is infectious meningitis, subarachnoid hemorrhage, or some other inflammatory condition."

"So meningeal irritation is an important finding when present, huh?"

"You bet it is," she said. "And that brings us to examination of the skull and spine, the fourth part of the 60-Second Ten-point Neuro Exam. Again, cervical manipulation is prohibited in the event of head trauma, but you should still make a thorough survey of the skull and spine, to the extent you can without moving the neck."

"What should the EMT look for?"

"In trauma cases you should look for scalp hematomas, lacerations, and contusions, with special attention to location. In patients with trauma and altered mental status, temporal contusions should alert you to the possibility of acute epidural hematoma."

"And what about examination of the spine?" I asked.

"Look for point tenderness, which can be produced by very light palpation of the spine."

"What does this tell the EMT?"

"In the case of elderly patients who fall," explained Brooks, "point tenderness over a vertebral body may help pinpoint the location of a compression fracture. When a flexion injury is involved, as in the case of a high-speed MVA, tenderness over the spine may direct you to the presence of an unsuspected vertebral body fracture."

I liked the systematic approach to neurologic assessment that Brooks was outlining. And she was good company, too. I couldn't think of a better way to learn about the 60-Second EMT.

"I think I'll have a slice of homemade apple pie," I said to Karen. "Would you like one, too?"

"Sure," she said. So I ordered the pie from the waitress.

"The fifth part of the 60-Second Neuro Exam is assessment of the patient's station and gait," continued Brooks. "The paramedic can elicit some very important information from this part of the exam. Of course, if the patient is nonambulatory or if ambulating represents some risk to the patient, this part of the exam should be deferred. Otherwise, inquire about and look for signs of falling to one side or another. This is usually caused by weakness of the side to which the patient is falling, and the most common disorder is a cerebral infarction, or stroke, on the side opposite the weakness. Naturally, if it's too risky to have the patient walk, observe his postural control while he is sitting in bed. If he falls to one side and can't maintain a sitting position, severe truncal weakness resulting from a stroke might very well be the culprit."

"This is a pretty comprehensive survey, isn't it?" I remarked.

Brooks pointed out, "It has to be, which is why Donnelly stresses evaluation of the twelve cranial nerves, the sixth component of the 60-Second Neuro Exam."

"There seems to be so much confusion about how to interpret abnormalities of the cranial nerves. I hope you can give me some guidelines," I said, as the waitress brought two steaming pieces of pie à la mode.

"All right," Brooks said. "Let's give it a try. The first cranial nerve, CN I, is the olfactory nerve. It conducts the sense of smell. People with seizure disorders can have olfactory hallucinations as a symptom, so it's important to be aware of this cranial nerve. The second cranial nerve, CN II, is the optic nerve, which is involved in visual perception. If patients can't see out of one eye, the CN II may be damaged. Remember, though, if a patient tells you it seems like one side of his visual field has been cut off but he is able to see half-fields in both eyes, there usually a problem in the occipital cortex. A stroke is the most common cause. The third (oculomotor), fourth (trochlear), and sixth (abducens) cranial nerves enable gazing in various directions. For example, if the eye is unable to look to the side, the CN VI is injured. If there is dysconjugate gaze (each eye is looking in a different direction), a brainstem lesion should be suspected. In fact, most gaze palsies—the inability to look down, up, or to the side—indicate a brainstem problem, usually a vascular event involving the vertebrobasilar system."

"Why is it important to distinguish a brainstem or peripheral lesion from a central lesion?" I asked.

The 12 Cranial Nerves

CN I → olfactory nerve—senses smell
CN II → optic nerve—visual perception
CN III → oculomotor nerve—directional gazing
CN IV → trochlear nerve—directional gazing
CN V → trigeminal nerve—facial sensory
CN VI → abducens nerve—directional gazing
CN VII → facial nerve—blinking reflex, all facial muscles
CN VIII → acoustic nerve—hearing
CN IX → glossopharyngeal nerve—innervates oropharynx structures
CN X → vagus nerve—innervates diaphragm, activates respiratory musculature
CN XI → accessory cranial nerve—innervates some muscles
CN XII → hypoglossal nerve—innervates tongue

Clinical Presentations of Acute Stroke

Abrupt onset of hemiparesis or monoparesis	Diplopia
	Ataxia
Sudden decline in state or level of consciousness	Quadriparesis
	Acute ataxia, vertigo, vomiting with or without headache (cerebellar stroke)
Cataclysmic headache	
Aphasia or dysarthria	
Visual loss (monocular or binocular); may be a partial loss of a visual field	

"Because, as a rule, brainstem problems are more serious. The consciousness center, the ascending reticular activating system (ARAS), is in the brainstem. So if a patient starts to pick off his cranial nerves, the prognosis is much worse and respiratory compromise may be down the road."

"I see," I said, as she continued.

"The fifth cranial nerve, CN V, is called the trigeminal, because it has three divisions. It's the large sensory nerve for the face and has a superior and inferior ophthalmic division as well as a mandibular branch. Absence of sensation in the face indicates that this nerve is compromised. Herpes zoster of the face usually affects one of the three divisions of the trigeminal nerve."

"Does the corneal reflex involve the fifth cranial nerve?" I inquired.

"Yes, actually it does," Brooks answered. "The sensory part of the corneal reflex is relayed by the ophthalmic division of the trigeminal nerve. The blinking reflex, however, requires an intact seventh, CN VII, or facial cranial nerve. This nerve is responsible for moving all the facial muscles: lifting eyebrows, smiling, and such."

"The difference between a 'central' and 'peripheral' seventh-CN deficit is quite important, isn't it?"

"Yes, and that's why Donnelly stresses this point in his 60-Second Neuro Exam."

"I'd like to hear his thinking about this part of the neuro exam."

"The seventh CN is often the most visible manifestation of a stroke in the region of the middle cerebral artery. A facial droop, which includes a lip and eyelid droop along with loss of the nasolabial crease, can be caused by a central lesion in the cerebral hemisphere or a peripheral lesion at the root of the seventh CN in the brainstem. In patients who have a visible facial droop and loss of skin folds on one side of the forehead, the EMT can distinguish between a peripheral and central lesion simply by asking the patient to lift his eyebrows and wrinkle the skin of his forehead."

"Why is this a useful maneuver?"

"Because each side of the forehead receives dual innervation from both cerebral hemispheres. Only one side has to be intact for a person to be able to wrinkle the skin. Therefore, if a patient is able to wrinkle his forehead, the peripheral seventh cranial nerve has to be intact, and the central control of the seventh on one side is gone. On the other hand, if the patient isn't able to wrinkle his brow, this means that the peripheral seventh CN is involved. As I mentioned, distinguishing between a peripheral and central seventh-CN palsy tells you whether the stroke is in the brainstem or the cerebral hemisphere."

"So it's really as simple as asking the patient to wrinkle the skin of his brow?" I asked.

"That's right," said Brooks. "Let's go on. The eighth cranial nerve, CN VIII, is the acoustic nerve, used for hearing. The ninth cranial, or glossopharyngeal, nerve CN IX, innervates structures in the oropharynx. The inability to swallow, or absent gag reflex, indicates that this nerve has been affected. The vagus, or CN X, innervates the diaphragm and activates the respiratory musculature. The eleventh, or accessory cranial, nerve, CN XI, innervates a number of muscles. Lack of ability to shrug the shoulders indicates that this nerve root has been compromised. The twelfth, or hypoglossal, nerve, CN XII, innervates the musculature of the tongue. The tongue will drift toward the side of the affected twelfth CN."

Speaking of tongues, mine was more than happy with the apple pie. "Did you like the pie?" I asked my instructor.

"Terrific," she said. "You think you've got those cranial nerves down?"

"Yep."

"Okay, that leaves the motor, sensory, cerebellar, and deep tendon reflexes—the last four components of the ten-point exam," she continued, without so much as a blink. Her cranial nerves were clearly intact. "The motor exam involves a brief survey of the patient's ability to move his extremities. The 60-Second EMT ought to pick up a hemiparesis this way. As you probably know, hemiparesis is usually caused by a stroke in the region of the middle cerebral artery, on the opposite side of course. In the event of trauma, inability to move the lower extremities may be the first sign of a spinal cord lesion. Loss of motor function is usually easier to assess than loss of sensory function, but the EMT should inquire about numbness and try to assess how objective or subjective this symptom is. Proprioception, or position sense, abnormalities should also be sought. For example, a wide-based gait is a sign of proprioception dysfunction. Cerebellar dysfunction is character-ized by loss of inhibition and gross intention tremor of involved extremities. Ataxia of the limbs, extremities that can't be adequately controlled, may indicate a cerebellar prob-lem. Chronic alcoholics can have cerebellar degeneration from alcohol toxicity.''

Deep tendon reflexes that are asymmetrical are a good first clue that neurologic damage of some sort has occurred.

"That leaves the deep tendon reflexes," I remarked.

"It does," Brooks said. "Deep tendon re-flexes that are asymmetrical are a good first clue that neurologic damage of some sort has occurred. In general, spinal cord lesions, or lower motor neuron lesions, will produce diminished reflexes. Hyperreflexia usually indicates a cerebral or upper-motor neuron problem. Finally, the presence of Babinski's reflex—the turning up rather than down by the great toe when the plantar aspect of the foot is stimulated with a scratch—is an ab-normal sign and indicates upper-motor neuron neurologic im-pairment. Well, that's the ten-point neuro exam. What do you think of it?''

"I think it's great," I said. "It really helps organize the EMT's approach to neurologic evaluation.''

"I know it seems like a lot to cover within the Golden Minute," she said. "But I've seen Jerry Donnelly complete this assessment in little more than a minute.''

"From what I've heard about Donnelly, that doesn't surprise me," I answered.

"The 60-Second Ten-point Neurologic Exam, of course, is only part of the key to understanding a patient's problem," pointed out Brooks. "The 60-Second Neuro Exam also emphasizes important aspects of the pa-tient's history. The abnormal physical signs uncovered by the 60-Second EMT are valu-able only if he can correlate them with com-

The abnormal physical signs uncovered by the 60-Second EMT are valuable only if he can corre-late them with common neuro-logic syndromes.

mon neurologic syndromes. Are you interested in hearing a brief overview of these? Jerry includes them in his 60-Second Neuro Assessment.''

"Absolutely," I said.

"Let's start with focal deficits," Karen began. "The most common cause of focal deficits, hemiparesis, central seventh nerve palsies, visual disturbances, focal seizures, etc., is thrombosis in a major cerebral vessel. Usually, the onset of the deficit is quite abrupt."

"What if the deficit appears and then shortly thereafter disappears?" I queried.

"That is called a transient ischemic attack, or TIA," Brooks explained. "It is still a serious problem because the blood supply to the affected area of the brain is very tenuous."

"When does cerebral artery thrombosis usually develop?" I asked. "In other words, what is the typical clinical picture?"

"It usually develops at night, during sleep, and the symptoms are perceived by the patient, or his family, upon wakening in the morning. As a rule, the patient falls asleep without a deficit but arises with a hemiparesis or some other focal deficit. Remember, as a rule, thrombotic cerebral infarction does not result in severe depression of consciousness unless the basilar artery system affecting the brainstem is involved. And seizures are also uncommon as the first manifestation of an acute thrombotic infarction."

"So what does it mean if your ten-point neuro exam reveals *both* a focal neurologic deficit, such as a hemiparesis, let's say, and a depressed level of consciousness?"

"In these situations, the EMT should suspect an expanding cerebral lesion, such as a hemorrhage that's causing compression of the brainstem. This is a key differential point. But it's important to ask about a history of diabetes as well, since hypoglycemia can also give you a picture of depressed mental status along with a

Common Causes of Seizures

1. Idiopathic
2. Alcohol or drug withdrawal
3. Reduction of or abrupt withdrawal of anticonvulsant drugs
4. Head trauma
5. Cerebral anoxia
6. Intracranial infection
   a. Abscess
   b. Subdural empyema
7. Intracerebral hemorrhage
8. Toxic-metabolic
   a. Hypoglycemia
   b. Hypocalcemia
9. Brain tumor
10. Subdural hematoma
11. Cortical vein thrombosis

focal problem. A postictal state can present this kind of picture, so the EMT should try to exclude a seizure disorder."

"In some patients, the stroke is caused by an embolism that's traveled to the brain rather than by a thrombosis, isn't it?"

"Yes, that's right," she confirmed. "Cerebral embolism can look just like a thrombotic stroke. In these patients, seizures are much more common. The presence of atrial fibrillation or the history of a recent myocardial infarction ought to point the EMT toward a cerebral embolism as the cause of the patient's neurologic deficit. In these individuals, a clot—a mural thrombus—has been dislodged from the wall of the heart and traveled to the brain, where it lodges in a major vessel and cuts off the blood supply."

I thought for a moment about the 60-Second Approach to Neurologic Assessment. The ten-point neuro exam—mental status, meninges, speech, skull and spine, station and gait, cranial nerves, and motor, sensory, cerebellar, and deep tendon reflexes—was useful for uncovering important physical findings. An understanding of the key neurologic syndromes—cerebral infarction, cerebral embolism, intracerebral hemorrhage, and metabolic disorders—would help direct the EMT toward likely causes of neurologic deficits uncovered by the exam. This approach was one I would find very useful in prehospital assessment.

I started to pick up the check. Before I could sneak a peek at the damage, Brooks reached over for the green piece of paper and said, "Listen, it's on me. Our crew just got a raise last week. And I feel like celebrating."

We walked out to the parking lot. Karen waved good-bye and I thought to myself, "Now there's a woman with all her neurons intact."

Drugs Used to Manage Cerebrovascular Emergencies

ANTICOAGULANTS

- Heparin is given 5,000 to 10,000 U IV (100 U/kg; loading dose should be reduced if patients >65 years of age), then 700 to 1200 U/h (10 to 20 U/kg/h) IV. The dose should be adjusted q 6 to 12 h until PTT is 1.2 to 1.4 × control. Warfarin (coumadin) therapy can begin immediately following heparin therapy and consists of an initial dose of 10 to 15 mg PO qD × 3d, followed by 4 mg PO qD in order to maintain PT time at 1.2 to 1.4 × control.

Continued

Drugs Used to Manage Cerebrovascular Emergencies—cont'd

ANTIHYPERTENSIVES

- Nifedipine capsules: 10 to 20-mg capsules, chew and swallow for rapid reduction of blood pressure (may also be used sublingually).
- Nitroprusside: A constant infusion should be tritrated gradually at an initial dose of 0.25 mcg/kg/min IV. The dose can be increased at increments of 0.25 mcg/kg/min up to a maximum of 10 mcg/kg/min.
- Labetalol: Begin with a 20-mg IV bolus (0.25 mg/kg), then 20 to 40-mg boluses IV q 10–15 min titrated to desired BP; this is followed by an infusion of 0.5 to 2 mg/min as required.

ANTICONVULSANTS

- Lorazepam: 4 to 8 mg IV at 1 to 2 mg/min slow IV infusion, or
- Diazepam: 5 to 10 mg IV at 1 to 2 mg/min slow intravenous infusion.

VASPOSPASM-REDUCING AGENTS

- Nimodipine: (60 mg) is administered every four hours, continuing treatment for up to 21 consecutive days after the initial event.

ANTI-PLATELET DRUGS

- Aspirin: (Dosage regimen still controversial): High-dose therapy (325 mg to 1300 mg/day) for prevention of TIA and stroke in nonvalvular atrial fibrillation versus low-dose aspirin therapy (30 to 80 mg/day) for prevention of TIA in patients with normal sinus rhythm.
- Ticlopidine

OSMOTIC AGENTS

- Mannitol: 1 to 2 g/kg of 20% solution given over 5 to 10 minutes and additional 0.5 to 1 g/kg every 4 to 6 hours will reduce ICP. It should be stressed that the use of mannitol is somewhat controversial. It represents only a temporizing measure and may lead to a rebound intracerebral incident

HUNT AND HESS CLINICAL GRADES OF SUBARACHNOID HEMORRHAGE

Grade 1: Asymptomatic or minimum headache or stiff neck.

Grade 2: More severe headache, stiff neck.

Grade 3: Confused or drowsy, may have mild hemiparesis.

Grade 4: Deeply stuporous, may have moderate to severe hemiparesis, early decerebrate signs.

Grade 5: Comatose.

EMERGENT MANAGEMENT OF SUBARACHNOID HEMORRHAGE

1. Correct any compromise of airway, breathing, or circulation.
2. Consult neurosurgery.
3. Reduce elevated blood pressure to pre-SAH levels.
4. Begin nimodipine 60 mg orally every four hours in patients Hunt and Hess Grades 1, 2, and 3.
5. Administer anticonvulsants if seizures occur.
6. Administer analgesics and sedatives as needed.
7. Consider emergency angiography, invasive hemodynamic monitoring, and early surgery in patients with aneurysmal SAH.

EMERGENT MANAGEMENT OF INTRACEREBRAL HEMORRHAGE

1. Correct any compromise of patient's airway, breathing, or circulation.
2. Consult neurosurgery promptly if need for surgical intervention is identified (e.g., cerebellar hemorrhage, acute hydrocephalus).
3. Do not treat hypertension urgently unless (a) the systolic and diastolic pressure exceeds 220 mm Hg or 120 mm Hg, respectively, on three repeated measurements made at 15-minute intervals; or (b) arterial dissection or cardiac failure has been identified.
4. If increased intracranial pressure is suspected, treatment with IV mannitol may help. In selected patients, hyperventilation of the lungs can be considered.

EMERGENT MANAGEMENT OF ACUTE ISCHEMIC STROKE

1. Correct any compromise of patient's airway, breathing, or circulation.
2. Do not treat hypertension unless (a) systolic blood pressure is >220 mm Hg or 120 mm Hg diastolic on three repeated measurements made at 15-minute intervals; (b) mean arterial pressure is greater than 140 mm Hg; or (c) patient is in danger of myocardial, aortic, or renal damage associated with elevated blood pressure.
3. Administer anticonvulsants if seizures occur.
4. Immediately consult neurosurgery if cerebellar infarction is diagnosed.

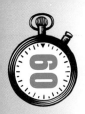

NEUROLOGY

I. Initial assessment and ABCs take priority over detailed assessment. If altered mental status is present, meticulous airway monitoring is a must!

II. The 60-Second Neurology Exam should include the following components:

A. **Mental Status**:

1. Orientation to person, place, and time.
2. Level of alertness.
3. Thought content: delirium (acute confusional state). Remember **MADCAP**:

   M for Medication reactions and Metabolic derangements (e.g., hypoglycemia).

   A for Alcohol and Anticholinergics.

   D for Dementia.

   C for Cardiac disorders and Cerebrovascular accident (CVA).

   A for Alterations in hemodynamic respiratory status, or environment.

   P for Pneumonia and associated sepsis.

B. **Speech:** presence or absence of aphasia or dysarthria.

C. Test for **Meningism** (pain and/or resistance to neck flexion but not to other neck movements). This will screen for the presence of meningitis and/or subarachnoid hemorrhage. **Note**: Omit the test for meningism in the setting of trauma.

D. Observe and palpate the **Scalp, Face, and Neck** for any sign of trauma.

E. Testing the **Cranial Nerves** will allow the very critical determination of any paralysis and/or sensory abnormalities as being of *central* as opposed to spinal or peripheral origin.

1. Test the visual fields (CN II).
2. Check the patient's extraocular movements (EOMS) (CNs III, IV, and VI).
3. Check for equal facial sensation (CN V).

4. Check the symmetry of the patient's facial muscles (CN VII).
   a. If face droops and patient cannot furrow brow symmetrically: a central lesion.
   b. If face droops and patient cannot furrow the brow on the same side: a peripheral seventh-CN palsy (e.g., Bell's palsy).
5. Check hearing to finger rub or watch tick (CN VIII).
6. Check for gag reflex (CN IX).
7. Check heart rate (CN X [vagus nerve]).
8. Check strength of shoulder shrug (CN XI).
9. Check tongue protrusion (CN XII).

F. **Motor Function**
   1. The most sensitive indicator of a hemiparesis, whether it is of central or of spinal origin, is the test for **Pronator Drift**:
      With the patient keeping his eyes closed, have him or her hold arms straight out in front with elbows unbent and palms up. A patient with a pronator drift will exhibit a rotation of the involved arm inward, with the arm drifting outward and down. This will show hemiparesis even in the presence of good muscle strength resting.
   2. Remember that **Priapism** (involuntary erection) in a patient is an index of spinal paralysis until proven otherwise.

G. **Sensory Function** to at least soft touch; if there is any question, assess sensation by another method, such as pinprick or temperature.

III. **60-Second Triage:**

A. **ALS**
   1. The **acute onset** of focal neurologic signs requires ALS assessment, treatment, and transport for the following reasons:
      a. What might appear to be a simple "stroke" may actually be an indirect side effect of a

myocardial event, such as an embolus from a mural thrombus as a result of an acute MI or atrial fibrillation.

b. A simple "stroke" may actually be due to a cerebral hemorrhage, which can decompensate at any time to involve severe intracranial hypertension with or without brain herniation. This will require aggressive airway management and controlled hyperventilation. Mannitol or steroids are usually avoided in the field unless long transport times are necessary. Research is being conducted that may show benefit from ultrapowerful steroid compounds given early for severe head injury.

c. It is well known that any acute neurologic event may induce cardiac dysrhythmias by a direct neurogenic mechanism.

d. The patient may actually be postictal with a "Todd's paralysis."

2. Any acute delirium (except perhaps caused by hypoglycemia or narcotics [see below]).

3. Coma, seizures, and altered mental status, as mentioned in previous modules.

B. **BLS**

1. Dementia with patient's inability to care for himself.

2. Subacute or chronic (slowly developing) syndromes (over the course of 4 weeks or more without a sudden change).

3. Clear-cut delirium—caused by hypoglycemia or narcotic intake clearly and completely reversed by $D_{50}W$ and naloxone, respectively—with transport times ≤ 20 minutes (see section on coma). Before giving D_{50}, try to determine BG level. D_{50} may be harmful to stroke patients. If in doubt, treat for hypoglycemia.

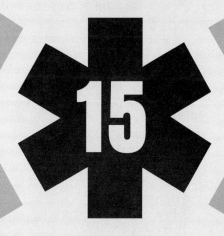

The 60-Second
Geriatric Assessment

very EMT I had met said that Larry Ashmead was one of the nicest guys around. From what Donnelly had told me, it was clear that Ashmead had a special place in his heart for old folks. Judging from his personal life, that concern began, as it often does, at home. Donnelly had filled me in on the details over the phone the night before my meeting with Ashmead.

Ashmead's parents retired several years ago. For much of the time they traveled extensively across America in their RV and, in general, lived a very active and productive life. Larry paid them regular visits, threw surprise anniversary parties for them, and included them in many of the social activities that were part of his own life. "He has a heart of gold," Donnelly confided, "and everyone knows it."

A few years ago, Larry's father died suddenly of a heart attack, leaving Larry's 82-year-old mother alone to fend for herself. Times got tough. Like other elderly people who lose a loved one, Mrs. Ashmead went through a period of severe depression. She required more and more of Larry's attention and emotional support . . . and she got it. From what I had heard, Larry was always there for her, giving above and beyond the call of duty. He even moved back home for a while, prepared meals for his mom, and involved her in community programs for the elderly. He packed her off to square dances, bought her a VCR so that she could watch movies at home, and placed her in a volunteer program at the local children's hospital. Thanks to his efforts, her spirits perked up considerably and she was soon on the road to recovery.

During that time, however, she developed some medical problems. Her doctor had started her on the beta blocker Tenormin® for angina, and gradually over a period of several weeks she became withdrawn and lethargic again. Larry suspected a medication reaction and called the doctor to give his opinion. As it turned out, he was right. His mother was, in fact, suffering from the side effects of Tenormin®. The doctor switched her to another beta blocker and she has been fine ever since.

Given his family circumstances, perhaps it is not surprising that Ashmead has developed a growing concern for the emergency health needs of the elderly. Actually, though, this has not always been the case. Geriatric medicine is a far cry from his original interest in prehospital care. As I learned, Ashmead started his EMT career riding with Donnelly, delivering prehospital care to the city's "knife and gun club." For a while, the excitement of the streets, .357 magnums, bullet wounds through the chest, and packets of white powder falling out of victims' pockets, turned Ashmead on. And no one could dispute, least of all Larry, that these experiences helped him mature into a seasoned, very skilled EMT. After resuscitating his twenty-eighth drug-related shooting victim in six months, however, Larry was ready for a change.

As Donnelly had explained during our telephone conversation the night before, "Ashmead developed a newfound appreciation for patients whose illnesses arose from *natural* causes." But that was only part of the reason for Ashmead's change of heart. It seemed to his friends that Ashmead's personal circumstances had kindled in him an interest in refining prehospital care for the elderly. Eventually, Larry requested a transfer to a district heavily populated by convalescent centers, retirement villages, and nursing homes. Ashmead has been providing prehospital care for the elderly patients in Gray Panther Estates for more than a year now. During this time, Donnelly has kept in contact, drawing heavily on Larry's expertise with the elderly to put together a 60-Second Assessment of Geriatrics for the 60-Second EMT program. It was my mission to find out what they had come up with.

I met Larry in front of his rig at the local teaching hospital. He was taking blood pressures of older folks who had come to a health fair at which the elderly were being screened for hypertension.

"Hello, Larry," I said. "I figured I'd find you helping out here." I looked around the converted parking lot, where hundreds of people were milling around booths. "Looks like a good cause," I offered.

"As good as they come," Larry replied.

He wrote some numbers down on a slip of paper and informed a woman who appeared to be in her sixties that she ought to see a doctor to have her blood pressure checked again. She said, "Thank you, young man," and walked off.

"You know, about 18% of Americans are over the age of 65," Larry began, as he smiled at the old-timers passing by. "That's about 30 million people. By the year 2000, one in every five, or about 20%, of Americans will be over the age of 65. It's estimated that there will be more than 14 million people over the age of 85!"

Those were impressive statistics.

"How does the 60-Second EMT fit into the picture?" I inquired.

"It's not just the 60-Second EMT," informed Larry. "It's the whole EMS community. Today, over 400,000 EMTs respond to more than 10 million emergency calls across the nation. About one third, or 3.3 million, of these calls involve patients over the age of 60. In some areas of the country, more than 60% of all ambulance "transports" are for the geriatric population. The numbers are growing. That's why Donnelly has developed a 60-second module tailored to this age group."

"Are you saying that the 60-Second Approach to Geriatric Assessment highlights specific issues involving the diagnosis and evaluation of the elderly?" I asked.

"That's right. Donnelly has developed two key components in the 60-Second Geriatric Exam. The first is the *geriatric awareness factor* (GAF), and the second is the *geriatric intervention factor* (GIF). You see, the 60-Second EMT has to be able to detect signs and symptoms of serious illness within the golden 'first' minute of contact with the patient. Donnelly's 60-second approach can help the EMT establish the severity of illness with a few crucial pieces of historical and physical information."

"Can you be more specific?" I requested.

"Sure. The GAF has to do with being aware, first, of the unique manner in which the elderly respond to nonurgent medical problems and, second, of the ways in which their signs and symptoms differ from younger patients in life-threatening disorders," explained Larry. "For example, when young people develop a viral pneumonia, an orthopedic problem, or get dehydrated from nausea and vomiting, they usually make an appointment with their physician. Illnesses such as these, at least in the younger population, usually can be treated in an outpatient setting. But it's different with old folks. The elderly frequently don't have the luxury of time. When they develop a 'nonurgent' problem—pneumonia, let's say—they may become debilitated very quickly and require ambulance transport."

> For the elderly, the spectrum of illness that demands EMT involvement is much broader than obviously life-threatening emergencies.

"So the 60-Second EMT has to be aware that for the elderly, the spectrum of illness that demands EMT involvement is much broader than obviously life-threatening emergencies," I said in an attempt to clarify the point.

"Yes, but that's only the first part of the GAF. The other point is that the EMT must be aware that signs and symptoms of life-threatening problems are frequently understated in the elderly. So, not only is the EMT transporting older patients with nonemergent problems, but he or she may be dealing with a very sick person whose outward symptoms or verbalization of the problem may not reflect how truly unstable he is. In short, the awareness factor means that the EMT has to keep both bases covered and establish priorities early in the patient encounter."

> **One-third of all heart attacks in the elderly occur without chest pain.**

"That sounds treacherous," I confessed.

"It is," Larry confirmed, "because symptoms in the elderly may not follow classical patterns. For example, one-third of all heart attacks in the elderly are 'silent,' or, in other words, occur without chest pain. Weakness, confusion, diaphoresis, nausea, vomiting, involuntary defecation, lethargy, or dyspnea may be the only presenting symptoms of a myocardial infarction. So extreme vigilance is required in elderly patients with these complaints. In particular, BLS units should not underestimate the importance of the symptoms. If there are any signs of hemodynamic instability or respiratory distress in an elderly patient with diaphoresis, vomiting, or shortness of breath, an ALS unit should be summoned immediately. This is especially true for any patient who has a past history of cardiac disease."

"I guess the GAF for cardiac emergencies in the older population encompasses a number of important issues. For example, the index of suspicion for cardiac ischemia is probably extremely high," I said.

"Exactly," warned Larry. "Without a constant awareness of the characteristic nature of older people's symptoms, the 60-Second EMT may misjudge life-threatening emergencies in this age group. Let me give you another example of what Donnelly stresses in the 60-Second Geriatric Exam. The middle-aged patient with cardiac angina commonly complains of chest pain, usually dull or pressure-like, radiating to the arm, shoulder, neck, or jaw. But in the elderly, these textbook signs and symptoms are frequently absent. In up to one-half of people over the age of 65, cardiac ischemia causes presenting dyspnea on exertion and progressive exercise intolerance. These symptoms in the geriatric age group are an anginal equivalent to chest pain in younger people. In other words, they suggest that the patient's deteriorating physical state is most caused by an inadequate supply of oxygen to the heart tissue, or cardiac angina. It's amazing to see Donnelly put these principles to work in the 60-Second EMT. The way he gets to the root of a patient's problem is magic."

"Did the two of you handle any cases in Gray Panther Estates that illustrate the importance of the GAF?"

"Lots of them," Ashmead remembered. "We were once called to see an 82-year-old woman complaining of weakness. On our arrival, the patient looked wiped out. While I took her vital signs, Jerry was making the best of his Golden Minute. It was clear from his line of questioning that Jerry knew weakness in a geriatric patient could mean any number of things. He spoke to her using clear diction, in a very reassuring tone. During the history, he gently placed his hand on her forearm and noted that she was diaphoretic.

" 'Any chest pain?' he inquired.

" 'No, none at all,' the woman said.

" 'Any nausea or vomiting?' Jerry asked next.

" 'No,' she said. By this time, I'd gotten the vital signs. Her heart rate was 110 with irregular beats, her respiratory rate was 24, and her blood pressure was 180/105."

"It sounds as if Donnelly hit a stone wall," I offered.

"That's what I thought, too, and I was prepared to just load and transport," Larry admitted. "But Donnelly was insistent on playing out the questions in his 60-Second Geriatric Exam. He asked, 'Are you short of breath, Ma'am?'

" 'No, not really right now,' the woman replied.

Then something clicked. It was as if the awareness factor kicked in, right on the spot. 'Have you noticed that you've been more short of breath lately, while walking or doing your usual activities?' Jerry inquired.

"Well, the woman looked at Donnelly in a way that said, 'I think this guy is on to something.' And then she said, 'As a matter of fact, I've been short of breath all week whenever I climb the stairs to my apartment. I've had to stop to catch my breath on the way to the grocery store, too. Funny, I've never had those problems before. Oh, and one more thing, I've been waking up in the middle of the night short of breath.' "

"With that kind of awareness, it's no wonder the 60-Second EMT works," I offered by way of praise for Donnelly.

"Now you see what I mean," Larry said. "In this case, Donnelly determined that the cause of the woman's weakness was cardiac angina. Even though she never had chest pain per se, she had dyspnea on exertion (DOE), which, in many elderly patients, is an anginal equivalent. So we hooked her up to the monitor, gave her nasal O_2 and, sure enough, she had ST elevation, suggestive of a myocardial infarction."

It was scary to think that elderly patients could have such atypical symptoms for common, life-threatening diseases.

"Larry, on the basis of the example you just gave," I said, "it sounds as if the EMT has to develop a whole new clinical language to assess elderly patients. It's almost like starting from the beginning."

"Maybe not a whole new language," Larry said, "but, as Donnelly points out in his 60-Second Geriatric Exam, a new awareness. That's what I've tried to stress."

"Does the geriatric awareness factor cover other problems besides cardiac diseases?" I asked.

"Absolutely," Larry responded. "Take, for example, falls by the elderly—a very important problem. Unfortunately, so many EMTs treat them all too casually. You know, the standard assessment goes something like this: 'Granny fell over the rug and broke her hip. Now, let's transport her to the hospital.' "

"Makes sense," I quipped.

"Yes, but this approach makes sense only if the EMT is sure that granny actually tripped over the carpet," emphasized Ashmead. "The elderly patient with a broken hip may very well have fallen because of GI bleeding, a cardiac arrhythmia, or a medication reaction. These are serious underlying causes that might be missed without the geriatric awareness factor Donnelly includes in his 60-Second Geriatric Exam."

"What does the awareness factor emphasize with respect to falls?" I inquired.

Larry explained, "The point is that the 60-Second EMT has to be aware that falls in the elderly are a result of both intrinsic (internal) and extrinsic (external) causes. In fact, 40% of all falls are caused by intrinsic factors such as cardiac syncope, stroke, dehydration, subdural hematoma, medication-induced postural hypotension, seizures, and GI bleeding. The 60-Second EMT works on the assumption that a fall as a result of extrinsic causes—tripping over a phone cord, slipping on a kitchen floor, or slipping on the steps—is a diagnosis of exclusion. In other words, serious intrinsic causes must be eliminated first through careful history-taking and physical exam. That's part of the 60-Second Geriatric Assessment."

The elderly patient with a broken hip may very well have fallen because of GI bleeding, a cardiac arrhythmia, or a medication reaction.

"But how do you establish intrinsic causes when the patient tells you—in fact, insists—that she fell because she tripped on the loose corner of a rug?" I asked. "What information does the EMT have to go on that causes him or her to suspect that something else is going on?"

Environmental Causes of Falls In The Elderly

OBSTACLE	MODIFICATION
	GROUND SURFACES
Highly polished or wet floors contribute to slipping.	In bathrooms, recommend nonslip glazed ceramic tile; nonslip adhesive strips placed on the floor next to tub, sink, and toilet; or indoor-outdoor carpet, which also reduces the risk of fall-related physical injury. Linoleum floors can be rendered slip-free with the use of slip-resistant floor wax and minimal buffing. Keep a nonskid floor mat by the kitchen sink to guard against a wet floor.
Thick pile carpets may lead to tripping.	Avoid thick pile or shag carpets. Recommend carpets of uncut, low pile.
Area rugs and mats may cause sliding falls.	Recommend that all rugs/mats have nonskid backing, or line back with double-faced adhesive tape.
Patterned carpets may lead to spatial misjudgment in persons with decreased depth perception.	Recommend plain, unpatterned carpets.
	LIGHTING
Poor environmental lighting may hide tripping/slipping hazards.	Provide increased lighting in high-risk fall locations (i.e., stairs, bathroom, bedroom).
Distracting glare from sunlight or lights shining on polished floors and unshielded light bulbs may impair vision.	Polarized window glass or application of tinted material to windows will eliminate glare without reducing light. Floor glare can be reduced by placing carpets on floor or repositioning light sources so that they do not shine directly on the floor.
	STAIRS
Poor lighting may contribute to stairway tripping.	Place light switches at top and bottom of stairs to avoid

Environmental Causes of Falls In The Elderly

OBSTACLE	MODIFICATION
	STAIRS—CONT'D
	traveling darkened stairways, or place night-lights by first and last step to provide visual cuing of steps. Placement of colored, nonslip adhesive strip will help define step edges.
Loss of balance on stairs may lead to serious falls.	Install handrails on both sides of stairs. Handrails should be round and set out far enough from the wall to allow for a good grasp.
	BATHROOM
Sink edges and towel bars may be used as assistive devices.	Replace towel bars with nonslip grab bars. Apply nonslip adhesive strips to the top of the sink to prevent slipping if grasped.
Transfer falls from low toilet seats.	Advise the use of elevated toilet seat and grab bars placed on the wall next to the toilet.
A slip and loss of balance may occur in the bathtub or shower.	Place nonslip adhesive rubber strips or mat with suction cups on tub floor. Install nonslip grab bars in and around the bathtub/ shower. Advise use of a shower chair and flexible hand-held shower hose for balance-impaired persons.
	BEDS
Transfer falls may occur from high/low beds.	A bed height of approximately 18 inches (from top of mattress to floor) will allow for safe transfers. Institutions can achieve a safe transfer height by using height-adjustable beds.
Poor sitting balance may lead to bed falls.	Bed mattress edges should be firm enough to support a seated person without sagging.

Continued

Environmental Causes of Falls In The Elderly

OBSTACLE	MODIFICATION
CHAIRS	
Trasnfer falls from low-seated chairs.	A chair height of 14 to 16 inches (from seat edge to floor) and armrests to provide leverage during rising/sitting will allow for safe transfers.
SHELVES	
Reaching or bending to retrieve objects from high or low shelves can lead to imbalance and falling.	Rearrange frequently used kitchen and closet items to avoid excessive reaching/bending. Shelf storage should be between a patient's hip and eye level. Encourage the use of hand-held reaching devices to obtain objects.

"That's a good question," agreed Ashmead. "The 60-Second EMT looks for any signs or clues that suggest intrinsic problems. Jerry and I were once called to see an elderly woman complaining of hip pain. When we arrived she was lying on the floor, incontinent of urine and in obvious distress from the painful discomfort in her hip. She seemed somewhat belligerent when Jerry asked what had happened.

" 'I was trying to get out of bed and tripped over the bedsheet when I stood up,' she declared with hostility.

" 'Did you black out?' Jerry asked.

" 'No, young man, I did *not* black out!' she shouted. 'For pity's sake, get me something for my pain. That hip is killing me!' "

"I guess you had to believe her story," I said.

"Most EMTs would have taken her explanation at face value, but the incontinence alerted Jerry, as did her belligerence, which seemed inappropriate under the circumstances," Larry explained. "As I took the vital signs, Jerry made a quick search around the room. He found three bottles of medicine. One of the bottles contained a diuretic, hydrochlorothiazide (HCTZ), that had been prescribed only three days earlier.

" 'Did you just start taking these?' Jerry asked.

" 'Yes,' the woman said, 'what business is it of yours?'

The Fall History	
A previous history of falling	Activity engaged in
Time of fall (hour of day)	Device utilization
Location	Presence of witness
Symptoms experienced	

"By this time I'd gotten her vital signs, and everything was normal except her blood pressure, which was 100/70 supine. When I told Donnelly the vital signs, he put the whole case together. He concluded she'd fallen because of orthostatic hypotension brought on by the new diuretic. He was absolutely right. We later learned that she also had a number of electrolyte abnormalities, including hypokalemia and hyponatremia, which contributed to her agitated behavior and which, it was surmised, might even have brought on a seizure that caused her incontinence. The bedsheet history was a total red herring."

It was clear from Ashmead's example that the 60-second assessment of geriatric patients requires the EMT to thoroughly search the environment. He has to pay special attention to physical findings and medications that could shed light on a patient's problem. In this case, the urinary incontinence, the recently prescribed antihypertensives, and the low blood pressure were the key pieces of the puzzle that pointed the EMT in the right direction. The search for extra information seemed especially important when there was reason to suspect that the patient's history might be inaccurate.

"I guess that when dealing with older patients, The 60-Second EMT is obligated to make a survey of the situation surrounding the event, especially since the patient can't always provide the needed data," I pointed out.

"You're getting my drift, now," Ashmead said with a satisfied ring in his voice. "And that brings me to the second part of the awareness factor in the geriatric exam: Histories given by elderly patients can be accurate, inaccurate, difficult to obtain, confusing, or misleading. For example, an elderly woman may *perceive* that she slipped on a carpet fragment when, in fact, she actually had a run of atrial fibrillation that made her woozy, causing her to fall. In such a case, the 60-Second EMT might note a rapid, irregular heart rate as part of the primary survey. Or, an elderly man may tell you he was walking down the street and got hit over the head with a hammer when, in reality, he may have had a spontaneous intracerebral hemorrhage that gave him the painful sensation of being hit on the head, after which he fell and lacerated his scalp. A blood pressure of 220/140 may alert the EMT to an intrinsic, rather than extrinsic, cause for the event. Finally, an elderly man may give you a history of passing out from the heat. In this situation, the 60-Second EMT would inquire about the presence of dark, tarry stools to confirm or rule out a diagnosis of GI bleeding. This is the kind of awareness that Donnelly demands of himself and of all EMTs who want to become proficient in caring for elderly patients."

Ashmead had made his point. And it was a good one. Some histories given by elderly patients are not reliable. But this isn't always the case. Some histories, and I know this from my own experience, are very accurate and provide critical information. I wanted some specific "pearls" and "pitfalls" for interviewing older patients.

I asked him directly, "When should the paramedic be suspicious about a history? How do we improve our chances of getting an accurate history? Any tips?"

"Tips?" Ashmead answered with a question. "That's what the 60-Second Geriatric Exam is all about. In fact, there are specific situations in which the 60-Second EMT should be on the lookout. In general, elderly persons weakened by illness may not be able to give an accurate history. They may be distracted by pain or discomfort. This is especially a problem when patients focus on only one source of severe pain, for example, hip pain. The pitfall is that patients may ignore discomfort elsewhere; for example, in the abdomen, head, or chest. Without a history of pain referred to these organ systems, the EMT might miss an abdominal aneurysm, chronic subdural, or myocardial infarction. When patients have hypoxemia, dementia, drug-induced confusion, toxicity from septicemia, or metabolic derangements, histories can also be compromised."

Communication and reassurance. These are the critical first steps that pave the way for geriatric evaluation in the prehospital setting.

"What if none of these underlying problems is present?" I inquired. "Is the EMT in the clear?"

"Not really," Ashmead continued. "A frequently encountered problem is the geriatric patient who is reluctant to give any history at all until trust and reassurance are established, which brings us

---

Remember . . .

Many elderly patients realize that if they leave home for a medical reason, they may not return.

Have patience and reassure your patients by doing the extras (lock the doors, tend to pets, etc.) whenever possible.

---

to two essential ingredients of the 60-Second Geriatric Assessment: communication and reassurance. These are the critical first steps that pave the way for geriatric evaluation in the prehospital setting. You've got to accomplish at least this much early in the Golden Minute."

"Does Donnelly have specific guidelines for the 60-Second Geriatric Exam?" I asked.

"We developed those early on." Ashmead nodded. "My experience in working with the elderly from Gray Panther Estates confirmed that without a reassured and trusting patient, it was almost impossible to obtain an accurate history and perform a worthwhile physical exam. Without both of these, the EMT can never arrive at a proper working diagnosis."

"What can the EMT do to improve communication with sick elderly patients?" I inquired.

"For starters, it's important to speak slowly and directly," informed Ashmead. "And, above all, be a good listener. Ask simple, straightforward questions. Patience is crucial."

"That's good advice," I confessed, "but what about those situations in which a patient's mental status is abnormal?"

"I'm so glad you brought that up," Ashmead said enthusiastically, "because you've just hit one of the major pitfalls in assessing elderly patients. The 60-Second EMT must always assume the elderly patient's mental status to be normal until he or she obtains direct testimony to the contrary from reliable bystanders, family members, or care providers."

"Why is that so critical?" I asked.

"Because the EMT can miss a potentially life-threatening problem if he doesn't follow this guideline. About a year ago, I saw Donnelly apply this principle in an elderly patient," Larry started, "and it literally turned my head around. We were called to see a 75-year-old man who had been mowing his lawn with a power mower and had fallen four feet over an embankment, landing on his head. When we arrived the patient was alert, able to give details of his fall, and had an obvious 5-inch laceration over his tem-

The 60-Second EMT

poral area. A BLS unit had arrived and one of the EMTs suggested to Donnelly that they transport the gentleman to the hospital."

"Did Donnelly agree?" I asked.

"Yes," Larry continued. "But as we carried the man to the ambulance by stretcher, Jerry started talking to him, and it became clear to Jerry that his thinking was a bit confused. The other EMT didn't seem to believe this was important and said to Donnelly, " 'Nothing to worry about, Jerry, he's an old guy and he's probably always a bit confused.' "

"Needless to say, that remark did not go over with Jerry. After a head injury, even the slightest impairment in mental status can be the first sign of a serious problem. Besides, the guy obviously had been alert enough to operate a power mower just a few minutes earlier. That's not something confused old people usually do. The long and short is that Jerry insisted on monitoring the patient's suspected altered mental status."

"So what finally happened?"

"Just what you'd expect," Larry beamed, obviously proud of his mentor. "The patient became sleepier and more confused on the way to the hospital. We had to intubate and transport him Code 3. The guy had an epidural hematoma, which was successfully evacuated by the neurosurgeon in the emergency department. The lesson I learned is that you must treat your older patients with the assumption that their baseline mental status is normal unless you have good evidence to the contrary. Remember, too, that so many acute problems in the elderly—infection, pneumonia, cardiac failure, COPD, drug reaction, dehydration, and others—present altered mental status as the first sign."

"Does Donnelly include any other assessment principles as part of the geriatric awareness factor?" I asked.

Medicine-induced problems are extremely common in this age group, especially in people taking three or more medications.

"I've covered most of them," Larry answered, "but, without question, one of the most important things the 60-Second EMT can do is take an accurate medication history from all geriatric patients encountered in the field. Medicine-induced problems are extremely common in this age group, especially in people taking three or more medications. Drug interactions are also important. In the elderly, it's important to be on the lookout for digoxin toxicity; orthostatic hypotension from antihypertensive medications; and for confusion from tranquilizers, narcotics, cimetidine, and anticholinergic drugs such as Benadryl®, tricyclic antidepressants, and certain sleeping pills. Be sure to ask if there have been any changes in medication dosages, especially in COPD patients, cardiac patients, and diabetics who might be prone to hypoglycemia. Of course, if there's any question as to whether a confused state may be caused by hypoglycemia, check the blood sugar and administer glucose immediately. Awareness of medication use in the elderly is a must.''

Larry's insights into Donnelly's 60-Second Geriatric Exam were invaluable. The GAF provided a good grounding for history-taking as well as a sound overall approach to elderly patients within the Golden Minute time frame. But I knew that there were pearls and pitfalls when it came to management of older patients, so I asked Larry to elaborate on them.

"As I mentioned earlier," began Ashmead, "the second part of Donnelly's 60-Second Geriatric Exam is the geriatric intervention factor, or GIF.''

"And what exactly is the GIF?'' I asked.

"The guiding principle of the GIF is that the approach to stabilizing elderly patients must be aggressive,'' explained Ashmead.

"Why is that emphasized?'' I queried.

"Because in older people, vital organ function may be significantly reduced as a result of the normal aging process or chronic illness,'' he explained. "There is limited reserve capacity in geriatric patients. What this means is that when elderly persons begin to deteriorate physiologically, they may be walking a fine line in terms of being able to provide oxygenation to tissues, or to maintain blood pressure or cerebral blood flow. Therefore, any delay in providing vital-organ (life) support or in treating a potentially life-threatening problem may have irreversible and devastating consequences in this age group.''

"Does the 60-Second Geriatric Assessment highlight specific issues?'' I asked.

"Yes, it does,'' answered Ashmead. "For example, elderly patients with acute GI bleeding who are hemodynamically unstable benefit from early administration of oxygen and IV fluids. These measures improve oxygenation of all tissues, including cardiac muscle, decrease the workload of the heart, and reduce cardiac irritability and the likelihood of life-threatening arrhythmias. Stroke volume also increases and normal organ perfusion can be maintained until the bleeding is controlled in the hospital. Without this intervention in the field, perfusion of vital organs may fall below tolerable limits, leading to sequential organ failure.''

Causes Of Unintentional Drug Toxicity In The Elderly

- Duplications
- Self-selection of drugs
- Taking prn drugs too frequently
- Automatic refills
- Omissions
- Pharmacy error
- Drug-induced confusion
- Recreational misuse

Causes Of Adverse Drug Reactions In The Elderly

- Multiple drug regimens
- Incorrect diagnosis
- Lack of compliance
- Poor OTC drug history
- Changes in drug metabolism
- Changes in drug effect (cardiac)
- Multiple physicians
- Generic versus trade names

Indications And Symptoms Of Possible Drug Toxicity

SELECTED DRUGS	REACTIONS
Chlorpropamide (Diabinese)	Hepatic changes, signs of congestive heart failure, bone marrow depression, seizures
Digitalis	Anorexia, nausea, vomiting, arrhythmias, blurred vision, other visual disturbances (colored halos around objects)
Furosemide (Lasix)	Severe electrolyte imbalance, impaired hearing and/or balance (ototoxicity), hepatic changes, pancreatitis, leukopenia, thrombocytopenia
Ibuprofen (Advil, Motrin, Nuprin)	Nephrotic syndrome, fluid retention, ototoxicity, blood dyscrasias
Lithium	Diarrhea, drowsiness, anorexia, vomiting, slurred speech, tremors, blurred vision, unsteadiness, polyuria, seizures
Methyldopa (Aldomet)	Hepatic changes, mental depression, nightmares, dyspnea, fever, tachycardia, tremors
Phenothiazine tranquilizers	Tachycardia, arrhythmias, dyspnea, hyperthermia, excessive anticholinergic effects
Procainamide (Pronestyl, Procan, others)	Arrhythmias, mental depression, leukopenia, agranulocytosis, thrombocytopenia, joint pain, fever, dyspnea, skin rash

Theophylline (Bronkodyl, Elixophyllin, others)	Anorexia, nausea, vomiting, GI bleeding, tachycardia, arrhythmias, irritability, insomnia, muscle twitching, seizures
Tricyclic antidepressants	Arrhythmias, congestive heart failure, seizures, hallucinations, jaundice, hyperthermia, excessive anticholinergic effects

Presenting Signs And Symptoms Of Drug Toxicity In The Elderly

- Acute delirium
- Akathisia
- Altered vision
- Bradycardia
- Cardiac arrhythmias
- Chorea
- Coma
- Confusion
- Constipation
- Fatigue
- Glaucoma
- Hypokalemia
- Orthostatic hypotension
- Paresthesias
- Psychic disturbance
- Pulmonary edema
- Severe bleeding
- Tardive dyskinesia
- Urinary hesitancy

Drugs Causing Orthostatic Hypotension

- Benzothiadiazides
- Bretylium
- Captopril
- Chlorisondamine
- Clonidine
- Tricyclic antidepressants
- Furosemide
- Guanethidine
- Guanidine
- Hexamethonium
- Hydralazine
- Iopanoic acid
- Levodopa
- Lidocaine
- Methotrimeprazine
- Methyldopa
- Methysergide
- Minoxidil
- Nifedipine
- Nitroglycerin
- Pentolinium
- Phenothiazines
- Phenoxybenzamine
- Prazosin
- Procarbazine
- Reserpine
- Thiothixene

Categories Of Adverse Drug Reactions In The Elderly

Primary Drug Reactions (One Drug–One Side Effect)

- Cimetidine psychosis
- Narcotic-induced respiratory depression
- Lidocaine psychosis
- Theophylline seizures
- Insulin reaction
- Chronic salicylism

Secondary Drug Interactions (Requires at Least Two Drugs to Cause Interaction)

- Sulfonylurea/sulfonamide
- Cimetidine/lidocaine
- Erythromycin/theophylline
- Indomethacin/propranolol
- Tricyclic antidepressant/alpha-sympatholytic

Drug Withdrawal Syndromes (Addictive and Nonaddictive Withdrawal)

- Beta-blocker withdrawal (angina)
- Calcium channel-blocker withdrawal (angina, hypertension)
- "Addictive drug" withdrawal syndromes (benzodiazepines, narcotics, etc.)

Tertiary "Extrapharmacologic" Effects (Measurable Only by Epidemiologic Studies)

- Falls caused by tricyclics, anxiolytics, and antipsychotics (short half-life versus long half-life agents)
- Traumatic injuries caused by drug-induced orthostatic hypotension

"I suppose, then, that the GIF applies to elderly patients with trauma as well," I remarked.

"Most definitely," Ashmead assured me. "Donnelly's geriatric awareness factor figures most prominently in elderly trauma patients. When the older person is a victim of injury, the clinical presentation can be misleading. For example, an elderly person with long-standing hypertension who is profoundly hypovolemic may have a normal blood pressure in the supine position. In fact, the heart rate may be normal if there is preexisting cardiac pathology or if the patient is taking a beta blocker for angina or high blood pressure. To avoid under-treatment of the elderly, the EMT must obtain a very detailed description of the mechanism of injury early in the Golden Minute. I might add, it is important not to be overaggressive in fluid replacement. You can push your patient over into pulmonary edema."

Obtain a very detailed description of the mechanism of injury early in the Golden Minute.

I began to appreciate how the GAF and the GIF work together in the overall approach to the geriatric patient—in particular, as it pertains to hemodynamic support.

"Any specific guidelines with respect to management of the airway?" I asked.

"Aggressive intervention is the key," said Ashmead. "Elderly overdose victims, for example, or older patients with a neurologic event such as intracerebral hemorrhage—in fact, all geriatric patients with a depressed gag reflex, cyanosis, and severe hypoventilation—need endotracheal intubation and positive-pressure ventilation in the field before they are transported. Not after they arrive in the emergency department with vomitus in their lungs and irreversible brain damage."

I was impressed with Donnelly's formulation of geriatric assessment, which focused on two key issues: *awareness and intervention.* And, when it came to taking a history, two key words: *trust and reassurance.* It was clear that Ashmead had devoted his professional life to the specific needs of geriatric patients and that the graying of our population would find him to be an invaluable asset to the medical community. He took a special pride in explaining the 60-Second Geriatric Exam, so much so that I suspected he had a vision for the overall function of EMTs in providing emergency health care for the elderly.

"Larry, if you had to summarize the role of the EMT in prehospital care of older people," I began, "what words of advice would you leave with me?"

"First, I'd strongly recommend that you get Donnelly's 60-Second Approach to Geriatric Assessment under your belt. If you learn the principles outlined in the GAF and GIF, you'll be way ahead of the game. But the other thing to recognize is that the EMT's role goes way beyond the Golden Minute. We're critical to the overall management plan of so many elderly patients."

"In what way?" I inquired.

"Perhaps the most important assistance the paramedic can offer the medical team is the in-home assessment and description of the older patient with altered mental status. This category of patient is especially difficult for the hospital team to diagnose and treat, because often the total picture is confusing as a result of the limited information available from the patient. The correct diagnosis may be delayed and appropriate care withheld because of insufficient information. To complicate matters, the older person often does not see a physician, or, for that matter, any other health care practitioner, on a regular basis. Records of previous and present medical illnesses may be grossly inadequate."

> **Talking with neighbors, friends, and family, as well as carefully inspecting the patient's home environment, may provide useful information necessary to make a diagnosis.**

"How does the EMT fit in?" I asked.

"Well, in these cases, the only useful information available about a patient's past medical history, environment, nutritional status, lifestyle changes, etc., may be what the EMT can gather at the scene. Talking with neighbors, friends, and family, as well as carefully inspecting the patient's home environment, may provide useful information necessary to make a diagnosis. In this light, EMTs and paramedics must look for medicines, poisons, signs of violent acts, physical abuse, neglect, or financial exploitation. They should ascertain that the elderly patient has not been denied access to appropriate medical care—one of the early signs of elderly abuse. They should evaluate the patient's ability to care for himself and self-administer medications as prescribed. Without these data, the hospital staff caring for the patient may be delayed several days in arriving at the correct assessment. For example, the simple observation that a patient is receiving a prescription from two or three different physicians may be the only clue that the cause of coma in an elderly person is a drug interaction. Such are important bits of information for which the 60-Second EMT is responsible."

Ashmead had given me a whole new slant on the 60-Second EMT. More important, he had inspired me to approach my elderly patients with a fresh set of insights drawn from Donnelly's 60-second program.

As he turned away to take the blood pressure of another elderly lady who had come to his booth I thought to myself, "Yeah, one of the nicest guys around . . . and one of the smartest."

GERIATRIC ASSESSMENT

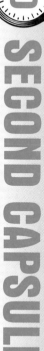

I. Remember the principles of the **geriatric awareness factor (GAF):**
   A. Elderly patients respond to nonurgent medical problems in a unique manner. They do not have the physiologic reserve of younger patients, and they become debilitated much more quickly. As a result, seemingly minor problems may become major ones.
   B. Signs and symptoms of life-threatening problems can vary in the elderly.
      1. Myocardial Infarction:
         a. Thirty-three percent occur without chest pain.
         b. Presenting symptoms can simply be sudden weakness, confusion, diaphoresis, nausea, vomiting, involuntary defecation, lethargy, or dyspnea.
         c. Any of the above symptoms occurring suddenly and without explanation in an older patient should be considered cardiac until proven otherwise and should be handled as an ALS call.
      2. Angina Pectoris can frequently appear only as a sudden deterioration in an elderly patient's exercise tolerance.
      3. Syncope in the elderly should always be an ALS call (see chapter on Syncope).
   C. Falls in the elderly merit special consideration of the GAF as well. Remember that 40% of falls in general have an **intrinsic** cause.
   D. In taking a history from a geriatric patient, keep in mind the principles of **communication** and **reassurance.**
   E. Always assume that the elderly patient's mental status has been normal until you obtain direct testimony to the contrary from reliable bystanders, family members, or care providers.

II. The **geriatric intervention factor (GIF):**
   A. The approach to stabilizing elderly patients must be aggressive.
   B. Remember from the GAF: there is limited reserve capacity in the geriatric patient.
III. One of the most important things the 60-second EMT can do in the evaluation of an elderly patient is to take an accurate **medication history** and do an **in-home assessment** of the patient's current living situation.
IV. **60-Second Triage:**
   A. **ALS** and **BLS** triage criteria generally do not differ for geriatric patients and younger patients.
   B. Exceptions to the above rule, where otherwise **BLS calls should probably be ALS calls** for elderly patients include:
      1. Syncope (with few if any exceptions).
      2. Falls, or any significant trauma of undetermined etiology.
      3. Sudden or subacute change in respiratory status.
      4. New or subacute change in mental status.
      5. Sudden nausea and vomiting of uncertain etiology.
      6. *Any* complaints of chest pain or discomfort.
V. 60-Second Medication Assessment:
   A. Powerful Medications:
      1. Antiarrhythmics.
      2. Antihypertensives.
      3. Antipsychotics.
   B. Polypharmacy.
   C. Compliance.

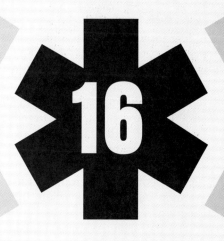

The 60-Second
Pediatric Assessment

ave Weimer had carved out a very special niche for himself in the EMS community. He was the training officer for a pediatric hospital–based ambulance company. Whenever a sick newborn needed transport from an outlying hospital to the pediatric intensive care unit, the suburban hospital staff always called Weimer's ambulance. When I had contacted Donnelly to ask him whom I might talk to about the 60-second approach to pediatric care, he strongly urged me to see Weimer. Apparently, Dave had a sixth sense with sick children, much like Larry Ashmead's special touch with geriatric patients. In fact, Donnelly was so impressed with Weimer's prehospital assessment skills in treating the pediatric age group that he had spent six weeks riding with Weimer, picking up pearls to incorporate in the 60-Second EMT Program.

The day I met Weimer, he had just finished a prehospital pediatric skills workshop, instructing EMTs on intubation techniques and cardiac arrest in children.

"Hello, Dave," I said, while he packed away the stylets and endotracheal tubes. "I really appreciate your taking the time to meet with me. Jerry said your specialized skills are quite in demand around here."

Weimer smiled. "That's true, but I'm always glad to share the approach Jerry and I developed for the 60-Second Assessment of the Pediatric Patient. It's tough to get access to good information about pediatric assessment in the field."

"Actually it is," I agreed. "You know, I just met with Larry Ashmead a few days ago to talk about Jerry's 60-second program."

"I know Ashmead, all right; he's topnotch," said Weimer.

"Well, then you probably know he specializes in the other spectrum of patients, the geriatric population," I said. "In his 60-second approach he discusses the assessment and triage of older patients in terms of geriatric awareness and intervention factors; he refers to them as the GAF and GIF. Did you and Donnelly develop a similar approach for pediatric patients?"

"As a matter of fact, yes," explained Weimer. "We decided to create some consistency in 60-second modules for these two patient populations. As you might expect, we developed a strategy called the *pediatric awareness factor* (PAF) and the *pediatric intervention factor* (PIF). As it relates to why they call Jerry Donnelly the 60-Second EMT, this strategy is what I would like to discuss with you today."

"I'm ready whenever you are."

"Okay, then, let's start at the beginning," said the EMT. "The basic premise Jerry stresses in his 60-second approach to prehospital care of pediatric patients is that children are not just 'small people.' Many paramedics, as well as physicians and nurses, seem to forget the special principles that apply to dealing with catastrophic illnesses in the pediatric age group."

> The basic premise of prehospital care of pediatric patients is that children are not just 'small people.'

"You're right. What makes it worse is that treating sick children really creates a lot of anxiety in EMTs," I pointed out.

"No doubt about that," he agreed. "It is truly frightening to be confronted with a critically ill child. Fundamental, though, to the PAF is the understanding that the principles of management still center around the ABCs of airway, breathing, and circulatory control.

"The 60-Second Pediatric Assessment presents a systematic approach to prehospital pediatric care. Specifically, it highlights the underlying causes of life-threatening illnesses in children. There are critical differences between children and adults as to precipitating factors. And, ultimately, this affects management."

"Where does Donnelly begin in his approach to pediatric care?" I asked.

"He starts with some basic principles about pediatric cardiac arrest," Weimer continued. "The important part of the PAF is to recognize cardiac arrest, or impending arrest, in the young child. In total arrest, the femoral and carotid pulses are absent. Auscultation reveals either absent heart sounds or marked bradycardia. Respirations are absent. Remember, in a neonate, for example, a heart rate of 60 is very abnormal and indicates impending cardiac arrest. Likewise, a respiratory rate of 12 in a neonate is dangerously close to complete apnea. The PIF demands that the EMT act quickly in these situations. As a rule, bradycardia is usually secondary to hypoventilation. Finally, it's always important to consider the possibility of hypothermia in a young infant."

I began to see why the PAF and PIF were so important to the 60-Second Assessment of the Pediatric Patient. There were critical differences in the interpretation of vital signs that would dictate prehospital management.

"As far as intervention goes, the resuscitation of an infant should be started in the field and continued regardless of the period of apnea or hope of survival," stressed Weimer. "Most experts would agree that in unusual circumstances, such as drowning, hypothermia, or electrical injury, resuscitation is indicated even if the period of apnea is prolonged."

> The resuscitation of an infant should be started in the field and continued regardless of the period of apnea or hope of survival.

"I assume the PAF stresses the unusual causes—unusual in the sense that they differ from those in the adult population—of cardiorespiratory arrest in infants. Is that right?" I asked.

"You're right, it does," Weimer said. "Sounds to me as if you've gotten a handle on the 60-Second EMT."

"I'd better by now," I confessed with wry amusement. "You're only the fifteenth person I've talked to trying to get to the heart of Jerry Donnelly's reputation as the 60-Second EMT."

"Great. So let's continue," Dave said. "The important causes of cardiac arrest in children include congenital heart anomalies, sepsis, hypovolemic shock secondary to gastrointestinal fluid loss, sudden infant death syndrome, foreign-body aspiration, drowning, and poisoning."

"This list is important for the EMT to keep in the back of his mind, isn't it?" I asked.

"Yes, and so is the fact that the majority of pediatric arrests are secondary to a respiratory arrest and that primary cardiac arrest is rare in children. I want to discuss foreign-body aspirations in a little while when I talk about respiratory arrest. But, for now, let's just say that it is critical in the PAF to take an accurate history so that the 60-Second EMT can rule in or rule out the possibility of a foreign-body aspiration as the cause of the child's respiratory arrest."

"What if you think the child has aspirated?"

"If aspiration is a strong possibility, vigorous attempts to remove the foreign body should be initiated within the Golden Minute," explained Dave. "In the case of an infant or small child, the primary resuscitator can hold the child prone over one arm and deliver strong back blows with the other hand. Remember, turning the patient completely upside down may force the object into the larynx, thereby completely occluding the airway. If noninvasive attempts are unsuccessful, direct visualization of the larynx should be performed so that the foreign body can be removed directly."

"I don't mean to change the subject," I said, "but EMTs get so little instruction in what to do if they're 'lucky' enough to deliver

APGAR Scoring System			
	0	1	2
Appearance (color)	Blue or pale	Body pink, extremities blue	Completely pink
Pulse (heart rate)	Absent	Slow (below 100 beats/min)	Over 100 beats/min
Grimace (reflex irritability to stimulation)	No response	Grimace	Cough or sneeze
Activity (muscle tone)	Limp	Some flexion of extremities	Active motion
Respiratory effort	Absent	Slow or irregular	Good crying

a baby. Does the PIF include a systematic approach to this kind of encounter?" I asked.

"As a matter of fact, it does," answered Weimer. "Remember that for neonates the management priorities are ABC and T. T stands for temperature because the newborn has very poor temperature control, and circulatory and respiratory status are entirely dependent on core temperature. If the infant you deliver is pink, crying, and has good movements (Apgar 8-10, see box above), use a clean, dry blanket to wrap the baby, keeping it close to the mother's perineum. Clamp the cord in two places about 10 inches from the infant; then cut the cord between the clamps."

"That's for the ideal situation," I pointed out. "What if the neonate isn't doing so well?"

Weimer explained, "If the infant's color is poor, it has a weak cry, and it is generally limp (Apgar 7 or less), hold oxygen tubing near the baby's face, keep it warm, and continue to stimulate respiration with suction. If respirations are inadequate or heart rate is less than 100, the EMT should assist with ventilation. CPR should be initiated if the heart rate is less than 80 beats per minute and if it is unresponsive to ventilatory control. Remember, too, if meconium—or what's called a 'brownish show'—is present in the upper airway, or an adequate open airway cannot be obtained, use a laryngoscope and a meconium aspirator."

"That's a nice basic guide, Dave," I said. "Now I'm ready to hear about Donnelly's approach to the infant with respiratory distress."

"Good, because that's where the pediatric awareness factor can really make a difference," he said. "There's no doubt that one of the most frightening problems an EMT can face is a child with breathing difficulties. For one thing, it's hard

Early, aggressive management of the airway can be lifesaving.

to quickly differentiate between serious and trivial causes of respiratory distress. And second, because opportunities for most EMTs and paramedics to become skillful and proficient in respiratory management of infants are limited, initiating invasive action is difficult. The key thing to remember, though, is that the primary cause of cardiac arrest in children is not cardiac disease but, rather, hypoxia, and that early, aggressive management of the airway can be lifesaving."

"How does Donnelly structure his approach to the child with respiratory compromise?" I inquired.

"The PAF stresses that this kind of problem can be caused by either upper- or lower-airway obstruction," said Weimer. "The most important signs and symptoms of upper respiratory tract obstruction are shortness of breath and stridor. Stridor may be either expiratory or inspiratory and tends to be most severe in laryngeal obstruction. As a rule, inspiratory stridor is associated with obstruction of the airway above the larynx or glottis, and expiratory stridor is associated with subglottic obstruction."

"Are there historical features of the case or signs and symptoms that can help with assessment?" I asked.

"Absolutely, and you should know that Jerry always uses a precise line of questioning and looks out for specific things when assessing such a patient," the EMT emphasized. "Important signs and symptoms for upper-tract obstruction include hoarseness, change in voice, difficulty swallowing food, oral secretions that can produce drooling, or loud wheezing."

"And what do you ask about at the scene?"

The most important signs and symptoms of upper respiratory tract obstruction are shortness of breath and stridor.

"A brief but accurate and precise history is the most important single contribution towards making an etiologic diagnosis of upper-airway obstruction," Weimer explained. "Without wasting a second, Donnelly will ask about the time of onset and activities surrounding the onset of respiratory problems, such as whether the child was eating or holding something in his mouth. And he'll want to know whether there were systemic symptoms such as fever, swollen neck glands, weakness, nausea, or vomiting."

"Exactly what does the exam consist of in patients who have clearcut obstruction?"

"That's where the pediatric intervention factor can offer a very specific set of guidelines," Weimer explained. "When examining a patient with upper airway obstruction, be brief but thorough. The EMT should examine the oral cavity, paying particular attention to the tongue and signs of inflammation or swelling in the mouth. The uvula, tonsils, and hypopharynx should be visible. But remember, unless the cause of an acute upper-tract obstruction is known, and it happens to be a foreign-body aspiration, care must be taken not to introduce any object into the airway or mouth for fear that the infant has epiglottitis."

"What's unique about airway obstruction caused by epiglottitis?" I asked.

"For one thing, it's a life-threatening emergency that can be made worse by overzealous management," he said. "Let me give you the clinical picture. Acute epiglottitis is characterized by the abrupt onset of rapidly progressive respiratory obstruction in a child usually two to eight years old. The clinical course commonly consists of the sudden onset of sore throat followed by pooling of secretions, drooling, and dysphagia. High fever is usually present, and stridor and dyspnea may interfere. Restlessness, cyanosis, and exhaustion can develop rapidly, and the patient's entire effort seems directed toward obtaining enough air, which is usually facilitated by quiet breathing rather than struggling. The child may attempt to lean forward in a 'tripod' position to help open her airway."

"And that's why the PIF offers some specific guidelines?" I asked.

"Exactly. Examination is best carried out with the patient in the sitting position, preferably on the mother's lap. EMTs should never try to introduce anything into a patient's mouth if the symptoms I just mentioned are present. The reason is that the child with epiglottitis usually stops breathing not from total obstruction of the airway, but as a result of complete exhaustion from the increased work of breathing and hypoxia. Consequently, when it comes to intervention, too much can be worse than just a little. Essential care includes positioning and administration of oxygen (blow-by is fine if placing a mask disturbs the child). Avoid upsetting the child in any way, and avoid IV attempts until arrival at the hospital."

"What if the child stops breathing en route?"

"Then immediately undertake assisted ventilation with a bag-valve mask. If the swollen epiglottis is making ventilation difficult, consider using an adult-sized bag with a child-sized mask. One EMT maintains a mask seal while another EMT ventilates. Avoid endotracheal intubation in the prehospital– or emergency department–setting. These patients should be intubated in an operating room by the most experienced person available. Remember that proper head and neck position is vastly important in children."

"So, as I understand it, the PIF in Jerry's 60-Second Pediatric Exam stresses the importance of minimizing agitation, physical activity, and oxygen consumption in an infant with obstruction caused by epiglottitis. The exam should be minimal once the diagnosis is established."

"That's correct," Weimer said. "The approach to assessment when a foreign-body aspiration is suspected is much different. As you know, children are particularly prone to aspirating objects such as beads or parts from small toys, which can become entrapped in the larynx. This problem usually occurs in children under the age of four. If a child is less than a year old, the foreign body is more likely to involve the lower airway. If the foreign body lodges in the upper airway at the larynx or above, the presenting symptoms are usually marked stridor and respiratory distress."

"Wheezing can help localize the object, right?" I asked.

"That's true, but, usually, wheezing is present only if the aspirated foreign body has passed the epiglottis and lodges in one of the mainstem bronchi. It may be unilateral, but because of the small chest size of the child, wheezing may be heard in both lung fields."

"How exactly does the 60-Second EMT differentiate between epiglottitis and aspiration?"

"Good question. Again, it's the history," he explained. "Aspiration of a foreign body should be considered in any child who has sudden onset of wheezing and inspiratory stridor without prior respiratory infection or history of wheezing events. As a rule, the diagnosis is made on the basis of a characteristic history."

"Once the EMT feels comfortable with this assessment, what does the PIF suggest?" I queried.

"For infants less than one year of age, only back blows and chest thrusts are recommended because of the concern for potential intraabdominal injury resulting from subdiaphragmatic thrusts used in the Heimlich maneuver," explained Weimer. "It's especially important to refrain from doing anything that might convert a partial obstruction into a complete one. This warning refers especially to the practice of turning very small children upside down and smacking them on the back to expel a foreign body that has already entered the tracheobronchial tree. Such a procedure is just as likely to cause a foreign body to lodge in the subglottic area as to expel it."

"That's useful information," I said. "Does the PAF include any more points regarding foreign-body aspiration?"

"As a matter of fact, yes," he said. "Donnelly stresses the importance of transporting patients when the EMT encounters the puzzling situation of a child who initially had signs of upper airway obstruction but, on the EMT's arrival, seems to have neither signs of ingestion nor symptoms of drooling, choking, or coughing that brought the child to the parent's attention in the first place."

"What does the 60-Second EMT do in this situation?"

"The best approach is to honor the history and to transport the patient, being careful to leave the child in the mother's or father's arms," explained Dave. "It's not unusual for these kids to be assessed in the emergency department, given a clean bill of health, and discharged, only to return with severe pneumonia and respiratory distress several hours later."

"What's the pitfall? When does this situation occur?" I asked.

"The EMT has to be especially cautious in peanut aspirations," continued Dave. "Initially, there may be complete relief from symptoms as the nut fragment moves distally down the bronchial tube. But over time, the peanut oil produces edema and severe local irritation leading to respiratory distress. Therefore, all children with peanut aspirations must be transported to the hospital regardless of how they look during your encounter."

Donnelly's 60-second approach to foreign-body aspiration tied together some loose ends for me, especially with respect to recognition, differentiation, and management. But I knew there were still other important pediatric conditions—croup and asthma— that lead to respiratory distress, and I wondered if Donnelly had devised a set of PAF and PIF criteria for them.

> Be especially cautious in peanut aspirations. All children with peanut aspirations must be transported to the hospital regardless of how they look during your encounter.

"What about croup and asthma?" I asked. "They're not quite as serious as the things you've been talking about, but they are part of the spectrum of diseases causing respiratory distress in children, aren't they?"

"Yes, they are," Dave said, "and fortunately, there are ways of differentiating these disorders from epiglottitis and aspiration. Croup, for example, is the term used to denote a hoarse, barking cough associated with difficult breathing. A one- to five-year-old with a history of a viral-like upper-respiratory illness that slowly progresses to stridor is an example of a patient with croup. These symptoms will usually be worse at night and when the child is lying down. Jerry stresses that the child with croup is in danger of asphyxiation caused by subglottic mucosal swelling and obstruction, but the danger is less imminent than with epiglottitis."

> **The EMT *can* alleviate respiratory distress in patients with croup with a cool, moist, humidified atmosphere.**

"Can the paramedic intervene when croup is suspected?" I inquired. "Or does the same 'hands-off' policy as in epiglottitis apply?"

"In fact, the EMT *can* alleviate respiratory distress in patients with croup and reduce such symptoms as stridor and shortness of breath," Dave answered. "Treatment includes a cool, moist, humidified atmosphere. The best approach is a face mask if the child can tolerate it, and if not, just let the cool mist stream into the patient's face. Keep in mind, though, that a small percentage of kids with croup may tire and require intubation."

"The same is true of asthma, isn't it?" I asked.

"Yes, but asthma is caused by reversible bronchospasm, which can be treated with albuterol inhalation or, if severe, epinephrine, 1:1000 solution at a dose of .01 ml/kg," pointed out Dave. "Remember, the history is the key to assessing a child with asthma. Inquire as to the various precipitators of bronchoconstriction, including allergies, irritants, exercise, emotional distress, and respiratory infections. Also remember to compare the severity of the current attack to previous incidents. The child who is markedly air-hungry, cyanotic, and has a prolonged expiratory phase with poor air exchange and *no* wheezing is in danger of imminent respiratory failure, and the EMT should be prepared to provide immediate airway care if needed."

"You know, Dave," I said, "I think the 60-Second Approach to Pediatric Assessment will really help organize my approach to kids with respiratory distress. I'm going to feel a lot more comfortable about this anxiety-provoking group."

"Terrific," Dave said. "That's what Donnelly was trying to do when he spent time sharing pediatric calls on my rig. But the PAF and PIF also apply to some other conditions that have to be approached much differently in the pediatric age group."

"What are some of the conditions?"

"Seizures in children, for one," explained Weimer. "As in adults, the treatment of an isolated seizure is primarily aimed at maintaining an airway and preventing the patient from injuring himself. If possible, keep the patient lying on his side to minimize the possibility of aspiration and clear all furniture and any potentially injurious objects away. As far as the PIF for seizures is concerned, *never* try to jam anything in the patient's mouth once the teeth are clenched. As soon as the tonoclonic phase of the seizure has abated, turn the patient on his side and continue to maintain the airway."

"And what about the PAF in pediatric seizures?" I inquired.

"The 60-Second EMT should be aware that two of the more common causes of status epilepticus, which is a series of rapidly recurring convulsions without any period of consciousness between, are withdrawal of anticonvulsant medications and hypoglycemia."

"Hypoglycemia?"

"That's right. A common error Donnelly and I detected in the field is that EMTs failed to give glucose to pediatric patients with seizures," Weimer pointed out. "Other causes of status epilepticus that are important to recognize include meningitis, electrolyte imbalance, and hypocalcemia, which is especially common in the newborn period."

"What about febrile seizures?" I inquired.

"The treatment is essentially the same, but it's important to know that simple febrile seizures rarely, if ever, produce status epilepticus. You have to consider other diagnoses when these occur, including epidural hematoma and surreptitious ingestion of drugs and other poisonings."

The 60-Second Pediatric Assessment offered a systematic approach to the assessment of two important pediatric emergencies: respiratory distress and seizures. The points Weimer made regarding intervention and awareness for these conditions proved that Donnelly's 60-second approach could encompass this special patient population.

> The 60-Second EMT should be aware that two of the more common causes of status epilepticus are withdrawal of anticonvulsant medications and hypoglycemia.

PEDIATRIC EMERGENCIES

I. Remember the principles of the **pediatric awareness factor (PAF):**
   A. As in the elderly, children and neonates have physiologic reserves different from those of adults; you need to be aware of these.
      1. The circulatory reserve is very small in infants. The loss of one unit of blood is sufficient to account for severe shock or death. Conversely, 500 ml of unnecessary fluid can result in acute fluid overload and pulmonary edema (an appropriate fluid challenge is 20 to 30 ml/kg).
      2. The neonate is particularly susceptible to hypothermia, and even a healthy newborn needs to be covered to prevent critical lowering of core body temperature.
      3. On the other hand, the brains of children have a much greater capacity than those of adults to survive conditions of no flow (as in a cardiac arrest), and they demonstrate a much greater plasticity in compensating for already established brain damage.
         For this reason resuscitative efforts need to be more aggressive and can be more prolonged than is normal for adults.
   B. Signs and symptoms of life-threatening problems can vary and be deceptive in the child and neonate:
      1. Remember that primary cardiac arrest in children is rare and usually is secondary to primary respiratory arrest or hypoxemia.
      2. An infant in arrest occasionally may be found held in a parent's arms with the parent totally unaware of the baby's crisis.
      3. A heart rate of <80 beats/min is critically low in a neonate and indicates the use of CPR if it does not improve with aggressive ventilatory efforts.

4. Respiratory distress in children also requires a different awareness:
   a. Foreign-body aspiration and upper-airway obstruction are more common and should always be considered.
   b. If the child with shortness of breath is also febrile, care must be taken not to place an instrument in the mouth or throat for fear of precipitating total obstruction in the case of epiglottitis.
5. Seizures are most often secondary to hypoglycemia and hypocalcemia (in the newborn).
6. Congestive heart failure may be present with various symptoms:
   a. There may be only tachypnea, tachycardia, diaphoresis, anorexia, cyanosis, or failure to thrive.
   b. Jugular venous distension (JVD) is rarely ever found in children's necks nor is increased capacitance of their hepatic vascular beds.
   c. Children and newborns may have only the symptom complex called **hypoxemic spells.** These are attacks of irritability, crying, hyperventilation, increased cyanosis, lethargy, or unconsciousness caused by intermittent right ventricular outflow and vasodilation found in congenital heart diseases such as tetralogy of Fallot.

II. Remember the **pediatric intervention factor (PIF):**
   A. The PIF is very similar to the Geriatric Intervention Factor (GIF). Because of the limited physiological reserves of children, interventions often need to be instituted more aggressively. But once initiated, more caution needs to be used in determining the endpoints of treatment (see previous discussion of limited circulatory reserves).

   Some cases, such as children with epiglottis, demand much more caution in beginning intervention.

B. Be aware of the differences in critical interventions:
   1. Endotracheal tube size: size of nostril or little finger, or the sum of 16 + age divided by 4.
   2. Cricothyrotomy should not be performed in a child under the age of eight.
   3. Avoid hyperextension of the neck in airway maneuvers.
   4. Begin CPR in neonates if the HR is <80 beats/min.
   5. Use suction for possible meconium aspiration because of the extremely heavy viscosity of the meconium.
   6. Use dextrose in all IVs of neonates because of their limited nutritional reserves.
   7. Keep a card of pediatric drug dosages handy at all times. Do not bother to try to memorize all the dosages unless you deal with a great many pediatric patients, but you should know the dosages of a few drugs and interventions that you may need to administer "in a pinch":
      a. Epinephrine: 0.01 mg/kg, 0.1 mg/kg for additional doses (cardiac arrest). Standard dose is first-line for bradycardia.
      b. Atropine: 0.02 mg/kg, 0.1 mg minimum. Now second-line for bradycardia.
      c. $D_{25}W$: 2 to 4 cc/kg.
      d. Valium: 0.2 mg/kg (0.5 mg/kg rectal).
      e. Defibrillation (if weight <50 kg): initial 2 joules/kg, double in subsequent attempts.
      f. Fluid challenge: 20 ml/kg.
   8. If IV access is difficult, remember the option of **intraosseous infusions.**
   9. $D_{25}W$ should be given for all pediatric seizures. Calcium should be considered in all seizures in neonates.

III. **60-second triage:**
   A. **ALS**: triage for pediatric patients, does not, in general, differ from that for adult patients. Possible exceptions in which otherwise-BLS patients should be ALS include:
      1. Any child with decreased responsiveness.
      2. Any out-of-hospital delivery, especially with a meconium show.
      3. Any motor vehicle accident in which an auto hits a child (auto-ped), regardless of the velocities.
   B. In general, scene times should be abbreviated for any critical or potentially critical pediatric patient.

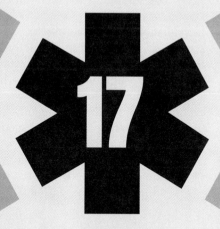

The 60-Second
Case Presentation
to the ED

Dr. John Duffens was the medical director for the paramedic protocol committee of the county in which Jerry Donnelly worked. Duffens was also an emergency department physician who oversaw the EMT training program at a large base station hospital. He and Donnelly had worked together on developing a logical, rational system for EMTs to use in presenting patients to physicians and nurses in the emergency department. Their goal was to develop an easily remembered approach that accounted for all the significant circumstances surrounding a patient's illness, the primary and secondary survey, emergency treatment administered, and the patient's subsequent disposition.

I met Dr. Duffens in his office, which commanded a sweeping view of the clinical facilities including the emergency department.

"Good morning, Dr. Duffens," I called, knocking gently on his door.

"C'mon in," Duffens said. "I've been expecting you."

Duffens was one of the new breed of emergency physicians. Part businessman, part clinician. Dressed smartly with a button-down shirt and tie, he appeared to be about 30 years old and very fit.

"Jerry told me you might be coming to see me. He says you're trying to figure out why they call him the 60-Second EMT. I can't think of a better learning experience."

"It's been a real eye opener so far," I confided.

"I bet," the physician said. "I'm particularly proud of the part of Donnelly's system I've had a chance to develop. Take a look at what's happening in this department right now."

Duffens pointed to the foyer, where patients were being transported through ambulance doors and wheeled into examination bays of the emergency department.

> An efficient and effective method for presenting patients to emergency personnel on the receiving end is a key feature in any EMS system.

"Every time our emergency physician or nurse receives an ambulance transport, critical information about that patient has to be communicated," began Duffens. "Even more important, the data have to be communicated efficiently and systematically. Emergency departments are generally overloaded and stressed. Consequently, an efficient and effective method for presenting patients to emergency personnel on the receiving end is a key feature in any EMS system. As you know, when you're passing off a patient to the emergency physician, there simply isn't enough time to stand around and ramble aimlessly about the circumstances surrounding the patient's illness. You've got about 60 seconds to tell the story and that's about it. In short, the EMT's presentation has to be concise, informative, and well organized."

"So how did you and Donnelly approach this problem of patient presentation?"

"The first thing we did was analyze the needs of the 60-Second EMT. We made a list of the critical data we felt needed to be communicated for every patient transport."

"And what did you come up with?"

"We came up with a 60-second presentation system we call 'RUSHED.'"

"'Rushed', huh? Well, that makes sense, and it's easy enough to remember," I offered. "If there's one thing we paramedics are, it's rushed whenever we present a patient."

"Each of the letters in RUSHED stands for a critical item of data that the 60-Second EMT should communicate to the emergency physician or nurse."

"Can you take me through it?"

"I'd be glad to," Duffens said. "The *R* in RUSHED stands for the *reason* that you were called to the scene. It also refers to the information that has come over the *radio* call from the dispatcher. Put simply, it stands for the reason for radio dispatch. This is the first information the EMT receives about the patient. For example, Donnelly will begin his presentation with something like, 'We were dispatched to see an 80-year-old woman who was found comatose at the bottom of the stairs in her apartment.' The *R* provides an overview of the patient's presentation. The *U* stands for *urgency* of the call and the degree of patient distress at the scene. The *S* stands for *scene assessment.* During this phase of the presentation,

---

Remember "RUSHED" when Presenting Patients to the ED

R = radio call and reason
U = urgency
S = scene assessment
H = history
E = evaluation
D = disposition, drugs and deployment of procedures

the EMT will recount any special features—prescription bottles, violation of passenger compartment in a motor vehicle accident, safety belt worn, environmental temperature, incontinence, etc.— that may provide critical information about the patient's problem. The *H* in RUSHED stands for the *history* offered by the patient or bystanders. The *E* stands for *evaluation* of the patient, including primary and secondary survey. And the *D* stands for *drugs, deployment* of stabilization procedures, and the *disposition* of the patient."

After thinking about it for a few moments, I could see the clarity and logic of the RUSHED approach. Radio, Urgency, Scene, History, Evaluation, Drugs, Deployment, and Disposition—these are key bits of information that have to be presented to emergency department personnel within the first minute of arrival in the emergency department.

"Dr. Duffens, can you recall a case that Donnelly presented using the RUSHED system?" I asked. "I'd be interested in hearing how the 60-Second EMT presents a patient using this method."

"No problem," Duffens said. "I remember the time we were called to expect a 68-year-old woman who was comatose and had a complex story. Upon arrival in the emergency department, Jerry painted the entire clinical picture using the RUSHED strategy. His presentation went something like this:

" 'We received a Code 3 call from central dispatch directing us to a 68-year-old white female [*R*] who was comatose with severe respiratory distress [*U*]. At the scene, the patient was found lying sideways in an unfilled bathtub and appeared cyanotic. Fresh vomitus was found on the floor and in the tub. An insulin syringe and bottle of regular insulin were found on the floor. Cardiac medications including digoxin and a diuretic were found on the bathroom sink [*S*]. The history was provided by the patient's daughter, who indicated that her mother had been depressed lately [*H*]. Evaluation revealed an elderly white female who was comatose with a blood pressure of 180/90, respirations of 32 and shallow, and heart rate of 120 and regular [*E*]. We put the patient on a backboard, stabilized the C-spine, started an IV, gave 10 L of O_2 by mask, drew a tube of blood, and administered 50 cc of $D_{50}W$, 2 mg naloxone, and 100 mg Thiamine at the scene. The patient's mental status improved dramatically. We transported, Code 3, to your facility [*D*].' "

It was evident that Donnelly had mastered the RUSHED approach from the way he had presented this complicated case. It was also clear to me that he had refined his 60-second approach so that a capsule presentation with all the pertinent data—from the radio call, to the history, to the final disposition—could be summarized in less than a minute. This was a system I planned to use the next time I was in the field.

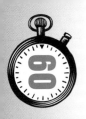

PRESENTATION OF PREHOSPITAL CASES TO EMERGENCY DEPARTMENT PERSONNEL

Use the **RUSHED** system for presenting relevant clinical data and histories when passing patients over to the emergency department nurses and personnel. Your verbal presentation should follow this sequence and include the following information:

Radio call and reason: Recount the information given by the radio dispatcher and the reason for being called to see the patient. Was an ALS or BLS unit called?

Urgency of patient's condition: Explain how stable or unstable the patient was upon your arrival. Be specific with respect to degree of respiratory distress, level of consciousness, extent of pain, and general condition.

Scene assessment: Describe relevant data at the scene. This would include a brief description of the patient's environment, if relevant; mechanism of injury, and how far the patient was from the vehicle if thrown from a car or motorcycle; general description of the environment: Was a windshield cracked? Was the passenger's compartment violated? Was a safety belt worn? In case of drug overdose, the EMT should note presence or absence of drugs, paraphernalia, etc.

History of patient's problem: This requires a brief description of events leading up to the patient's medical deterioration.

Evaluation of patient: Communicate the pertinent positive and negative features of the primary and secondary survey.

Disposition, drugs, and deployment of procedures: Inform the emergency physician or nurse as to what drugs were administered, what procedures were deployed (i.e., intubation, fluid administration, etc.), and final disposition of the patient.

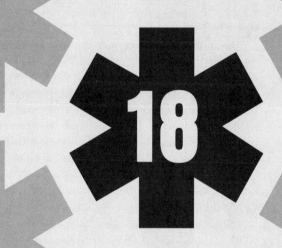

The 60-Second EMT:
Epilogue

After visiting with Jerry Donnelly's co-workers, I felt confident that I knew what the 60-Second EMT was really all about. But the only way to be sure that I had learned my lessons was to put theory into practice. That's exactly what I did one night while working on a BLS unit in Donnelly's district.

We were called to see an older person who reportedly had tripped over a telephone cord at home and was complaining of hip pain. We arrived on the scene and found an elderly woman pinned between her bed and the wall. I took a thorough history that followed the principles outlined in the 60-Second Assessment of Syncope. I learned that the woman had lost consciousness just before her fall. On physical exam, I noted that the patient had been incontinent of urine; she was diaphoretic and appeared confused. Her pulse was irregular. Her right leg was shortened and externally rotated. The patient continued to focus on her hip pain and had no other complaints.

On the basis of this assessment, which took just over a minute, I was concerned that this was something more than a typical fall caused by an extrinsic problem. The incontinence, diaphoresis, confusion, and syncopal episode suggested the possibility of a myocardial infarction. Even though the woman did not complain of chest pain, I suspected that the pain in her hip was diverting her attention from any other source of discomfort. Perhaps at her age the typical symptoms of myocardial infarction might be absent.

I immediately placed her on oxygen and called an ALS unit for transport. Within 8 minutes a unit arrived. The paramedics walked into the room with a stretcher and I could not believe my eyes. One of the medics was Jerry Donnelly! I wasn't sure if he recognized me. I gave him a 60-second presentation and offered my assessment of the patient's problem. Jerry nodded, seemed pleased, and hooked up the cardiac monitor. The patient had ST-T wave segment elevation and multiple PVCs.

"I think you're absolutely right," Donnelly said. "It looks as if she very well may have had a myocardial infarction followed by a syncopal episode and, perhaps, even a seizure. Who knows, she may have had a run of ventricular tachycardia. Good work. It's a good thing you called us."

"Thanks," I said.

"By the way," he continued, "where did you learn to assess patients so quickly and efficiently?"

It was clear that he did not remember me.

"I learned it from your co-workers," I said. "I am the person who came to talk to you about the 60-Second EMT a few months ago."

"Oh, that's right," he said with a twinge of embarrassment. "I must apologize. I can't recall your name. What is it?"

"Roxanne," I said.

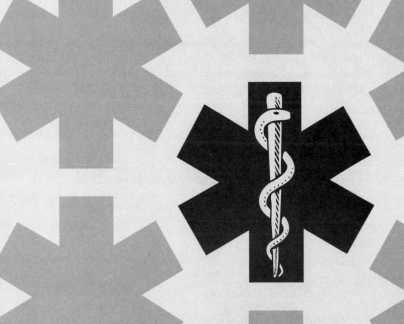

Appendix:
60-Second Rapid
Assessment Modules
for ABCs

The following assessment and intervention modules are included for "heat of battle" reference when urgent stabilization of the ABCs is required. Pull-out cards of these modules are available at the back of the book.

60-SECOND CLEAR AIRWAY MODULE A

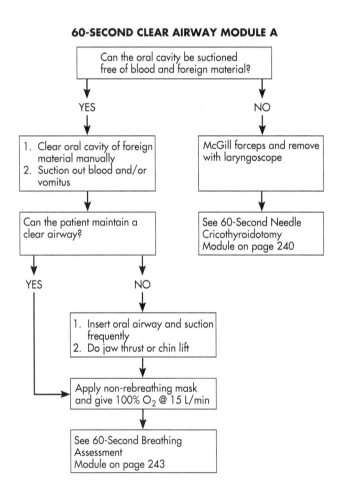

60-SECOND CLEAR AIRWAY MODULE B

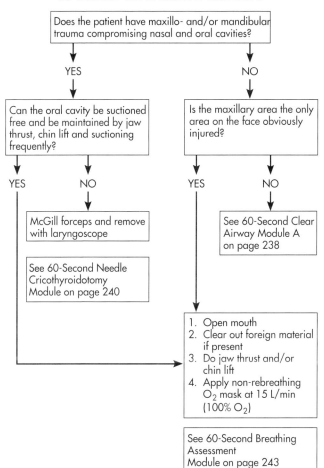

Does the patient have maxillo- and/or mandibular trauma compromising nasal and oral cavities?

YES

NO

Can the oral cavity be suctioned free and be maintained by jaw thrust, chin lift and suctioning frequently?

Is the maxillary area the only area on the face obviously injured?

YES   **NO**

YES   **NO**

McGill forceps and remove with laryngoscope

See 60-Second Clear Airway Module A on page 238

See 60-Second Needle Cricothyroidotomy Module on page 240

1. Open mouth
2. Clear out foreign material if present
3. Do jaw thrust and/or chin lift
4. Apply non-rebreathing O_2 mask at 15 L/min (100% O_2)

See 60-Second Breathing Assessment Module on page 243

60-SECOND NEEDLE CRICOTHYROIDOTOMY MODULE

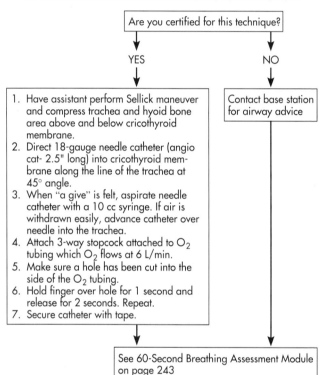

Are you certified for this technique?

YES

NO

1. Have assistant perform Sellick maneuver and compress trachea and hyoid bone area above and below cricothyroid membrane.
2. Direct 18-gauge needle catheter (angio cat- 2.5" long) into cricothyroid membrane along the line of the trachea at 45° angle.
3. When "a give" is felt, aspirate needle catheter with a 10 cc syringe. If air is withdrawn easily, advance catheter over needle into the trachea.
4. Attach 3-way stopcock attached to O_2 tubing which O_2 flows at 6 L/min.
5. Make sure a hole has been cut into the side of the O_2 tubing.
6. Hold finger over hole for 1 second and release for 2 seconds. Repeat.
7. Secure catheter with tape.

Contact base station for airway advice

See 60-Second Breathing Assessment Module on page 243

60-SECOND BREATHING DIFFICULTY ASSESSMENT MODULE

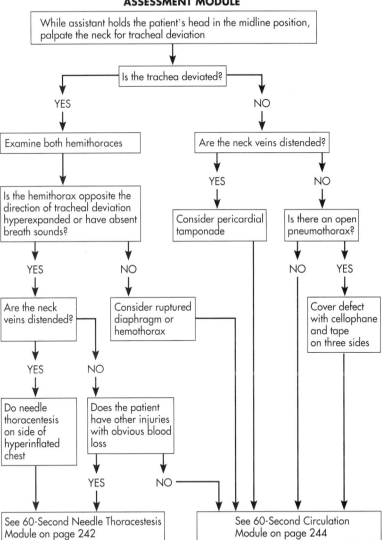

While assistant holds the patient's head in the midline position, palpate the neck for tracheal deviation

Is the trachea deviated?

YES → Examine both hemithoraces

Is the hemithorax opposite the direction of tracheal deviation hyperexpanded or have absent breath sounds?

    YES → Are the neck veins distended?

        YES → Do needle thoracentesis on side of hyperinflated chest

        NO → Does the patient have other injuries with obvious blood loss

            YES → See 60-Second Needle Thoracestesis Module on page 242

            NO → See 60-Second Circulation Module on page 244

    NO → Consider ruptured diaphragm or hemothorax

NO → Are the neck veins distended?

    YES → Consider pericardial tamponade

    NO → Is there an open pneumothorax?

        NO

        YES → Cover defect with cellophane and tape on three sides

See 60-Second Needle Thoracestesis Module on page 242

See 60-Second Circulation Module on page 244

60-SECOND NEEDLE THORACENTESIS MODULE

1. Identify 2nd intercostal space by locating angle of Louis on sternum and moving fingers laterally along rib on side of suspected tension pneumothorax to mid-clavicular line.
2. Direct 18-gauge needle catheter (4-6" long) perpendicular to 3rd rib until rib is encountered, then move tip of needle superior to 3rd rib and into thorax. (A rush of air should occur.)
3. Slide catheter over needle into pleural cavity and attach to tubing and Heimlich valve or tubing and finger of rubber glove cut to make a Heimlich valve.
4. Secure with tape without kinking catheter and tubing.

See 60-Second Circulation Module on page 244

60-SECOND BREATHING ASSESSMENT MODULE

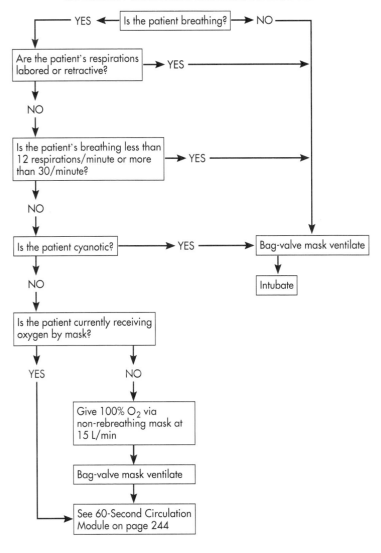

60-SECOND CIRCULATION MODULE

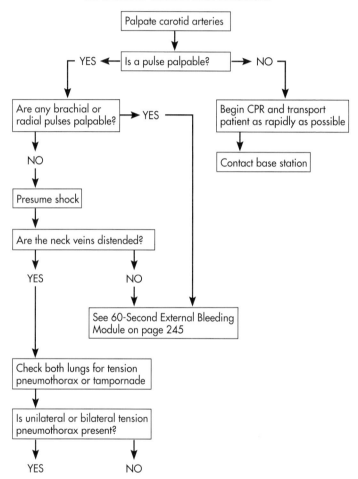

60-SECOND EXTERNAL BLEEDING MODULE

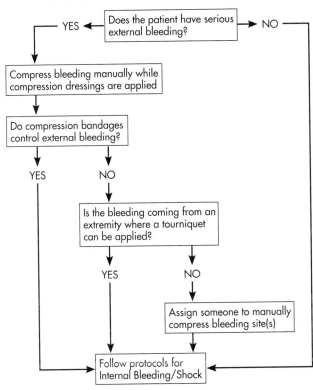

60-SECOND IV MODULE

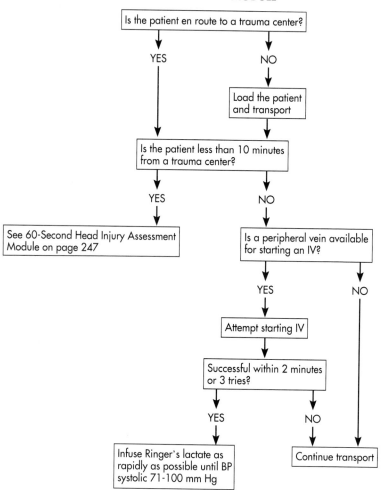

60-SECOND HEAD INJURY ASSESSMENT MODULE

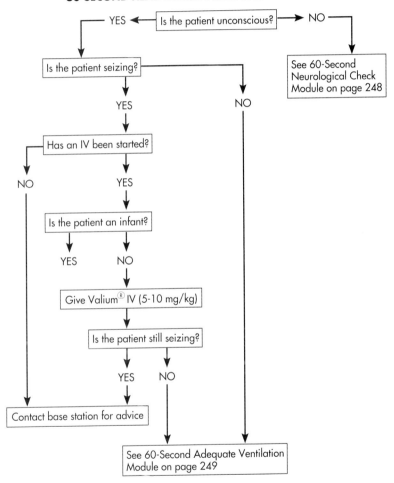

60-SECOND PUPIL AND NEUROLOGICAL CHECK MODULE

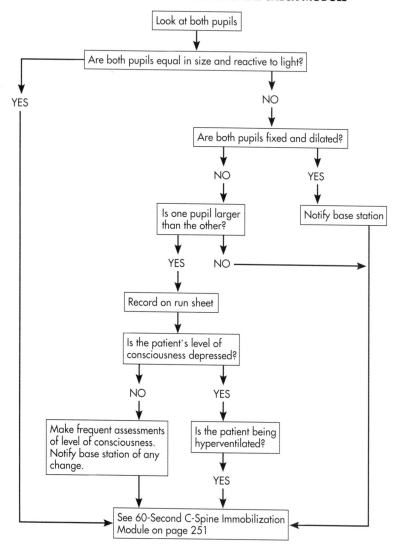

60-SECOND ADEQUATE VENTILATION MODULE

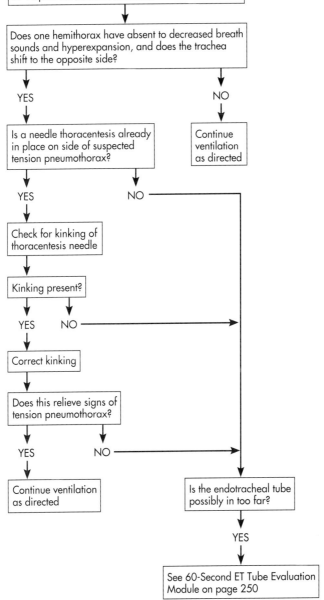

1. Listen for breath sounds in both hemithoraces.
2. Look at chest wall movement with each inspiration.
3. Palpate for tracheal deviation.

Does one hemithorax have absent to decreased breath sounds and hyperexpansion, and does the trachea shift to the opposite side?

YES — Is a needle thoracentesis already in place on side of suspected tension pneumothorax?

NO — Continue ventilation as directed

YES — Check for kinking of thoracentesis needle

NO

Kinking present?

YES — Correct kinking

NO

Does this relieve signs of tension pneumothorax?

YES — Continue ventilation as directed

NO

Is the endotracheal tube possibly in too far?

YES

See 60-Second ET Tube Evaluation Module on page 250

60-SECOND ET TUBE EVALUATION MODULE

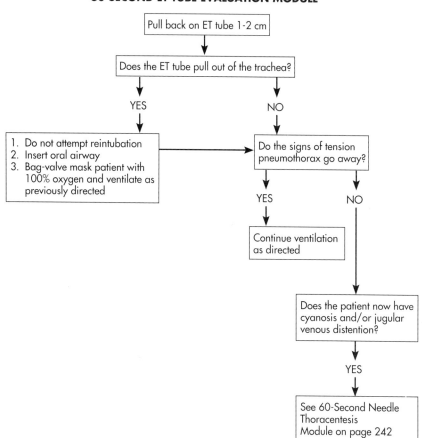

C-SPINE IMMOBILIZATION

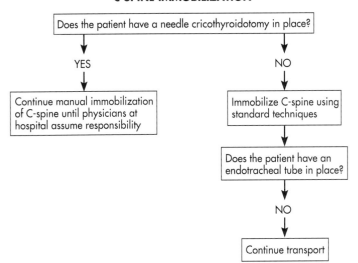

Does the patient have a needle cricothyroidotomy in place?

YES   NO

Continue manual immobilization of C-spine until physicians at hospital assume responsibility

Immobilize C-spine using standard techniques

Does the patient have an endotracheal tube in place?

NO

Continue transport

Index

60-SECOND CLEAR AIRWAY MODULE A

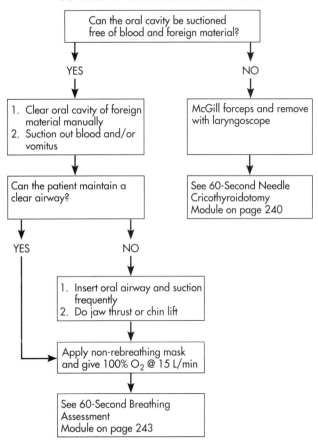

Can the oral cavity be suctioned free of blood and foreign material?

YES

1. Clear oral cavity of foreign material manually
2. Suction out blood and/or vomitus

Can the patient maintain a clear airway?

YES **NO**

1. Insert oral airway and suction frequently
2. Do jaw thrust or chin lift

Apply non-rebreathing mask and give 100% O_2 @ 15 L/min

See 60-Second Breathing Assessment Module on page 243

NO

McGill forceps and remove with laryngoscope

See 60-Second Needle Cricothyroidotomy Module on page 240

60-SECOND CLEAR AIRWAY MODULE B

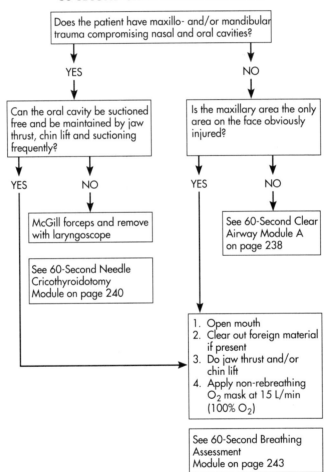

Does the patient have maxillo- and/or mandibular trauma compromising nasal and oral cavities?

YES

Can the oral cavity be suctioned free and be maintained by jaw thrust, chin lift and suctioning frequently?

YES / **NO**

McGill forceps and remove with laryngoscope

See 60-Second Needle Cricothyroidotomy Module on page 240

NO

Is the maxillary area the only area on the face obviously injured?

YES / **NO**

See 60-Second Clear Airway Module A on page 238

1. Open mouth
2. Clear out foreign material if present
3. Do jaw thrust and/or chin lift
4. Apply non-rebreathing O_2 mask at 15 L/min (100% O_2)

See 60-Second Breathing Assessment Module on page 243

60-SECOND NEEDLE CRICOTHYROIDOTOMY MODULE

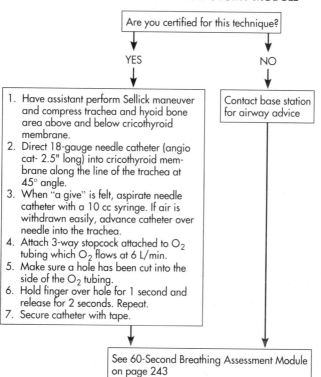

Are you certified for this technique?

YES

NO

1. Have assistant perform Sellick maneuver and compress trachea and hyoid bone area above and below cricothyroid membrane.
2. Direct 18-gauge needle catheter (angio cat- 2.5" long) into cricothyroid membrane along the line of the trachea at 45° angle.
3. When "a give" is felt, aspirate needle catheter with a 10 cc syringe. If air is withdrawn easily, advance catheter over needle into the trachea.
4. Attach 3-way stopcock attached to O_2 tubing which O_2 flows at 6 L/min.
5. Make sure a hole has been cut into the side of the O_2 tubing.
6. Hold finger over hole for 1 second and release for 2 seconds. Repeat.
7. Secure catheter with tape.

Contact base station for airway advice

See 60-Second Breathing Assessment Module on page 243

60-SECOND BREATHING DIFFICULTY ASSESSMENT MODULE

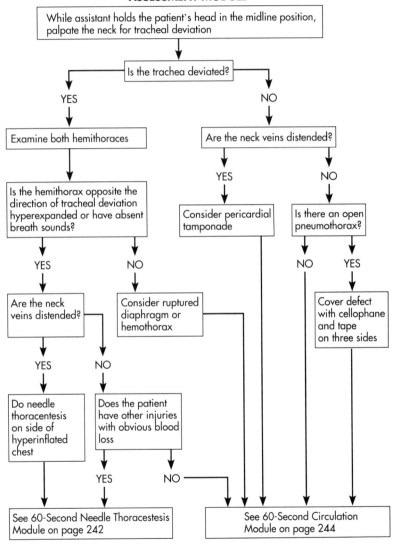

While assistant holds the patient's head in the midline position, palpate the neck for tracheal deviation

Is the trachea deviated?

YES → Examine both hemithoraces

Is the hemithorax opposite the direction of tracheal deviation hyperexpanded or have absent breath sounds?

YES → Are the neck veins distended?

YES → Do needle thoracentesis on side of hyperinflated chest → See 60-Second Needle Thoracestesis Module on page 242

NO → Does the patient have other injuries with obvious blood loss

YES → See 60-Second Needle Thoracestesis Module on page 242

NO → See 60-Second Circulation Module on page 244

NO → Consider ruptured diaphragm or hemothorax → See 60-Second Circulation Module on page 244

NO → Are the neck veins distended?

YES → Consider pericardial tamponade → See 60-Second Circulation Module on page 244

NO → Is there an open pneumothorax?

NO → See 60-Second Circulation Module on page 244

YES → Cover defect with cellophane and tape on three sides → See 60-Second Circulation Module on page 244

60-SECOND NEEDLE THORACENTESIS MODULE

1. Identify 2nd intercostal space by locating angle of Louis on sternum and moving fingers laterally along rib on side of suspected tension pneumothorax to mid-clavicular line.
2. Direct 18-gauge needle catheter (4-6" long) perpendicular to 3rd rib until rib is encountered, then move tip of needle superior to 3rd rib and into thorax. (A rush of air should occur.)
3. Slide catheter over needle into pleural cavity and attach to tubing and Heimlich valve or tubing and finger of rubber glove cut to make a Heimlich valve.
4. Secure with tape without kinking catheter and tubing.

↓

See 60-Second Circulation Module on page 244

60-SECOND BREATHING ASSESSMENT MODULE

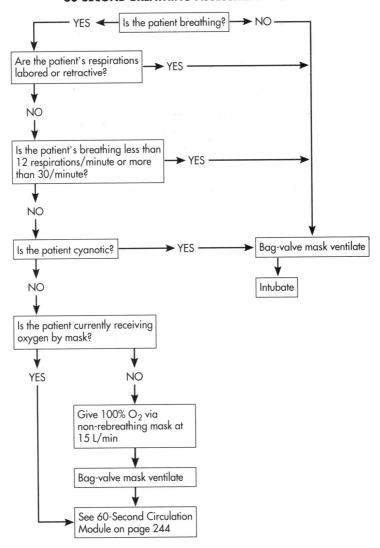

60-SECOND CIRCULATION MODULE

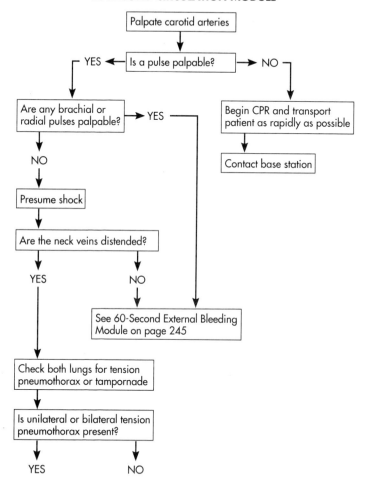

60-SECOND EXTERNAL BLEEDING MODULE

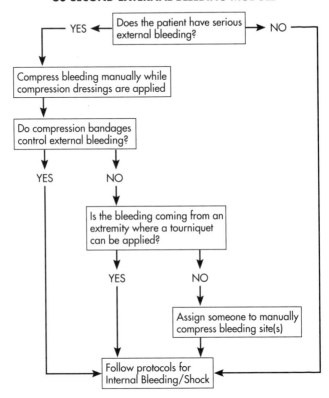

60-SECOND IV MODULE

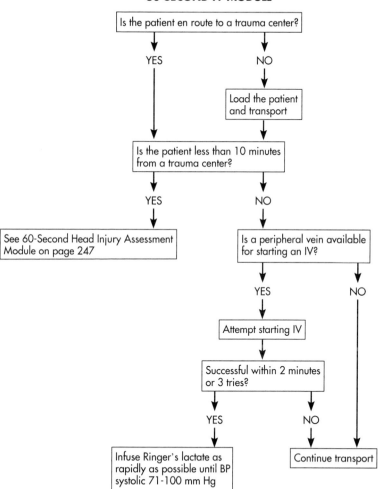

60-SECOND HEAD INJURY ASSESSMENT MODULE

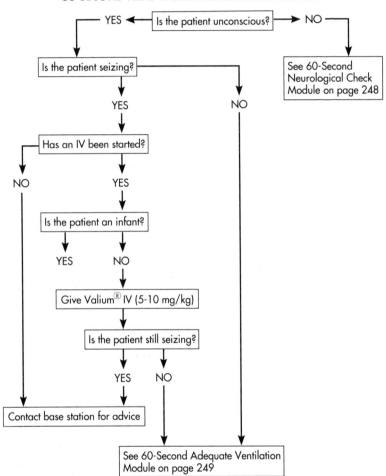

60-SECOND PUPIL AND NEUROLOGICAL CHECK MODULE

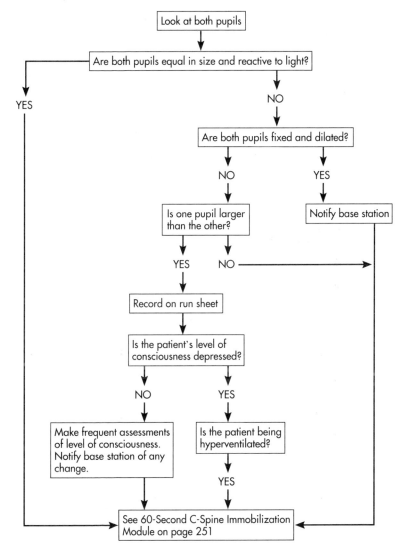

60-SECOND ADEQUATE VENTILATION MODULE

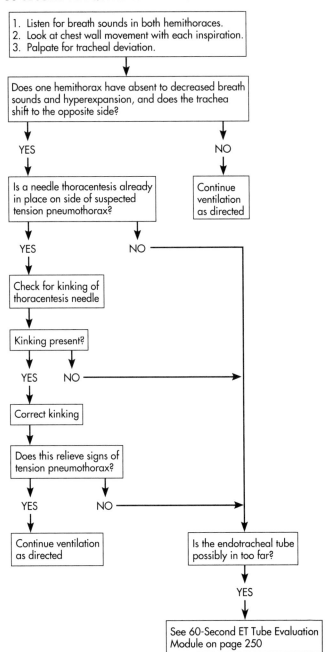

1. Listen for breath sounds in both hemithoraces.
2. Look at chest wall movement with each inspiration.
3. Palpate for tracheal deviation.

Does one hemithorax have absent to decreased breath sounds and hyperexpansion, and does the trachea shift to the opposite side?

YES

NO

Is a needle thoracentesis already in place on side of suspected tension pneumothorax?

Continue ventilation as directed

YES

NO

Check for kinking of thoracentesis needle

Kinking present?

YES

NO

Correct kinking

Does this relieve signs of tension pneumothorax?

YES

NO

Continue ventilation as directed

Is the endotracheal tube possibly in too far?

YES

See 60-Second ET Tube Evaluation Module on page 250

60-SECOND ET TUBE EVALUATION MODULE

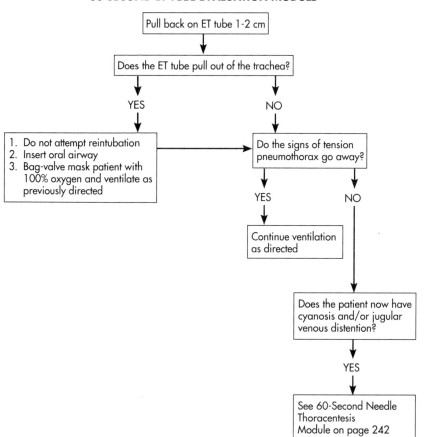

C-SPINE IMMOBILIZATION

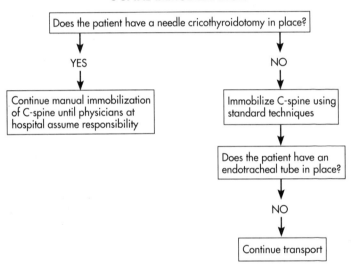